Metal Ions in Life Sciences Series

Volume 26

Metal-Containing Molecules and Nanomaterials:
From Diagnosis to Therapy

Guest Editor

Ana de Bettencourt-Dias
Department of Chemistry,
University of Nevada,
Reno, NV 89557, USA

Series Editors

Astrid Sigel, Helmut Sigel
Department of Chemistry
Inorganic Chemistry
University of Basel
St. Johanns-Ring 19
CH-4056 Basel
Switzerland
astrid.sigel@unibas.ch
helmut.sigel@unibas.ch

Eva Freisinger, Roland K. O. Sigel
Department of Chemistry
University of Zürich
Winterthurerstrasse 190
CH-8057 Zürich
Switzerland
freisinger@chem.uzh.ch
roland.sigel@chem.uzh.ch

CRC Press
Taylor & Francis Group
Boca Raton London New York

CRC Press is an imprint of the
Taylor & Francis Group, an **informa** business

Cover illustration: The figure was taken from Chapter 6 by permission of Rebeca L. Fernandez, Vanessa J. Lee, and Marie C. Heffern

First edition published 2024
by CRC Press
2385 NW Executive Center Drive, Suite 320, Boca Raton, FL 33431

and by CRC Press
4 Park Square, Milton Park, Abingdon, Oxon, OX14 4RN

CRC Press is an imprint of Taylor & Francis Group, LLC

Library of Congress Cataloging-in-Publication Data
Names: de Bettencourt-Dias, Ana, editor.
Title: Metal-containing molecules and nanomaterials : from diagnosis to therapy / edited by Ana de Bettencourt-Dias, Professor, University of Nevada, Reno, NV, USA.
Description: First edition. | Boca Raton : CRC Press, 2024. |
Series: Metal ions in life sciences | Includes bibliographical references and index. |
Identifiers: LCCN 2024000842 (print) | LCCN 2024000843 (ebook) |
ISBN 9781032422145 (hardback) | ISBN 9781032422169 (paperback) |
ISBN 9781003361756 (ebook)
Subjects: LCSH: Metals in medicine. | Metals—Therapeutic use.
Classification: LCC RS431.M45 M48 2024 (print) | LCC RS431.M45 (ebook) |
DDC 615.9/253—dc23/eng/20240325
LC record available at https://lccn.loc.gov/2024000842
LC ebook record available at https://lccn.loc.gov/2024000843

ISBN: 978-1-032-42214-5 (hbk)
ISBN: 978-1-032-42216-9 (pbk)
ISBN: 978-1-003-36175-6 (ebk)

ISSN 1559-0836   e-ISSN 1868-0402

DOI: 10.1201/9781003361756

Typeset in Times New Roman
by codeMantra

About the Editors

Ana de Bettencourt-Dias received her 'licenciatura' (MS equivalent) in Technological Chemistry from the University of Lisbon in 1993 and her 'Dr. rer. nat.' (PhD equivalent) in Inorganic Chemistry from the University of Cologne in 1997 with Prof. Thomas Kruck. In her graduate work, she isolated new titanium complexes as single-source precursors for the chemical vapor deposition of TiN thin layers. She joined the group of Prof. Alan Balch at UC Davis in 1998 as a Gulbenkian post-doctoral fellow, where she studied the electrochemistry and structure of fullerenes and endohedral fullerenes. In 2001, she joined the faculty at Syracuse University and started her work on luminescent lanthanide ion complexes. She moved to the University of Nevada, Reno (UNR) as an associate professor in 2007 and was promoted to professor in 2013. Her research centers on light-emitting compounds and coordination chemistry of the f block of the periodic table. She served on the editorial advisory board for Inorganic Chemistry from 2013 to 2015, has been on the editorial advisory board for Comments on Inorganic Chemistry since 2016, is a managing member of the editorial board of the *Journal of Rare Earths* since 2014, and has been on the editorial board of Inorganics since 2022. She was program chair of the 2011 and conference chair of the 2014 Rare Earth Research Conference, organizes symposia of the Division of Inorganic Chemistry at the national meetings of the American Chemical Society, and was the 2019 Chair of the Division of Inorganic Chemistry of the American Chemical Society. She served as the Associate Vice President for Research at UNR from 2015 to 2019. She returned to being a full-time faculty member in July 2019 and is now the Susan Magee & Gary Clemons Professor of Chemistry. She received the 2006 Science & Technology Award of the Technology Alliance of Central New York, is a 2021 Fellow of the American Chemical Society, and is a 2022 Fellow of the American Association for the Advancement of Science. In 2022, she was named UNR Foundation Professor and was recognized as UNR Researcher of the Year in 2023.

Astrid Sigel has studied languages; she was an Editor of the *Metal Ions in Biological Systems* (*MIBS*) series (until Volume 44) and also of the *Handbook on Toxicity of Inorganic Compounds* (1988), the *Handbook on Metals in Clinical and Analytical Chemistry* (1994; both with H. G. Seiler and H.S.), and the *Handbook on Metalloproteins* (2001; with Ivano Bertini and H.S.). She is also an Editor of the *MILS* series from Volume 1 on, and she co-authored more than 50 papers on topics in Bioinorganic Chemistry.

Helmut Sigel is Emeritus Professor (2003) of Inorganic Chemistry at the University of Basel, Switzerland. He is a Co-editor of the series *Metal Ions in Biological Systems* (1973–2005; 44 volumes) as well as of the Sigels' new series *Metal Ions in Life Sciences* (since 2006). He also co-edited three handbooks and published over

350 articles on metal ion complexes of nucleotides, amino acids, coenzymes, and other bio-ligands. Together with Ivano Bertini, Harry B. Gray, and Bo G. Malmström, he founded (1983) the International Conferences on Biological Inorganic Chemistry (ICBICs). He lectured worldwide and was named Protagonist in Chemistry (2002) by *Inorganica Chimica Acta* (issue 339). Among Endowed Lectureships, appointments as Visiting Professor (e.g., Austria, China, Japan, Kuwait, UK), and further honors, he received the P. Ray Award (Indian Chemical Society, of which he is also an Honorary Fellow), the Alfred Werner Award (Swiss Chemical Society), and a Doctor of Science *honoris causa* degree (Kalyani University, India). He is also an Honorary Member of SBIC (Society of Biological Inorganic Chemistry).

Eva Freisinger is Associate Professor of Bioinorganic Chemistry and Chemical Biology (2018) at the Department of Chemistry at the University of Zürich, Switzerland. She obtained her doctoral degree (2000) from the University of Dortmund, Germany, working with Bernhard Lippert, and spent 3 years as a postdoc at SUNY Stony Brook, USA, with Caroline Kisker. Since 2003, she has performed independent research at the University of Zürich, where she held a Förderungsprofessur of the Swiss National Science Foundation from 2008 to 2014. In 2014, she received her *Habilitation* in Bioinorganic Chemistry. Her research is focused on the study of plant metallothioneins, with an additional interest in the sequence-specific modification of nucleic acids. Together with Roland Sigel, she chaired the 12th European Biological Inorganic Chemistry Conference (2014 in Zürich, Switzerland) as well as the 19th International Conference on Biological Inorganic Chemistry (2019 in Interlaken, Switzerland). She also serves on a number of Advisory Boards for international conference series; since 2014, she has been the Secretary of the European Biological Inorganic Chemistry Conferences (EuroBICs) and is currently co-Director of the Department of Chemistry. She joined the group of Editors of the *MILS* series from Volume 18 on.

Roland K. O. Sigel is Full Professor (2016) of Chemistry at the University of Zürich, Switzerland. In the same year, he became Vice Dean of Studies (BSc/MSc), and in 2017, he was elected Dean of the Faculty of Science. From 2003 to 2008, he was endowed with a Förderungsprofessur of the Swiss National Science Foundation, and he is the recipient of an ERC Starting Grant 2010. He received his doctoral degree *summa cum laude* (1999) from the University of Dortmund, Germany, working with Bernhard Lippert. Thereafter, he spent nearly 3 years at Columbia University, New York, USA, with Anna Marie Pyle (now Yale University). During the 6 years abroad, he received several prestigious fellowships from various sources, and he was awarded the EuroBIC Medal in 2008 and the Alfred Werner Prize (SCS) in 2009. Between 2015 and 2019, he was the Secretary of the Society of Biological Inorganic Chemistry (SBIC), and since 2018, he has been the Secretary of the International Conferences on Biological Inorganic Chemistry (ICBICs). His research focuses on the structural and functional role of metal ions in ribozymes, especially group II introns, regulatory RNAs, and on related topics. He is also an Editor of Volumes 43 and 44 of the *MIBS* series and of the *MILS* series from Volume 1 on.

Historical Development and Perspectives of the Series

*Metal Ions in Life Sciences**

It is an old wisdom that metals are indispensable for life. Indeed, several of them, like sodium, potassium, and calcium, are easily discovered in living matter. However, the role of metals and their impact on life remained largely hidden until inorganic chemistry and coordination chemistry experienced a pronounced revival in the 1950s. The experimental and theoretical tools created in this period and their application to biochemical problems led to the development of the field or discipline now known as *Bioinorganic Chemistry, Inorganic Biochemistry*, or more recently also often addressed as *Biological Inorganic Chemistry*.

By 1970, *Bioinorganic Chemistry* was established and further promoted by the book series *Metal Ions in Biological Systems* founded in 1973 (edited by H.S., who was soon joined by A.S.) and published by Marcel Dekker, Inc., New York, for more than 30 years. After this company ceased to be a family endeavor and its acquisition by another company, we decided, after having edited 44 volumes of the *MIBS* series (the last two together with R.K.O.S.) to launch a new and broader minded series to cover today's needs in the *Life Sciences*. Therefore, the Sigels' new series is entitled

"Metal Ions in Life Sciences".

After publication of 22 volumes (since 2006), we are happy to join forces from Volume 23 on in this still growing endeavor with Taylor & Francis, London, UK, a most experienced Publisher in the *Sciences*.

The development of *Biological Inorganic Chemistry* during the past 40 years was and still is driven by several factors; among these are (i) attempts to reveal the interplay between metal ions and hormones or vitamins, etc.; (ii) efforts regarding the understanding of accumulation, transport, metabolism, and toxicity of metal ions; (iii) the development and application of metal-based drugs; (iv) biomimetic syntheses with the aim to understand biological processes as well as to create efficient catalysts; (v) the determination of high-resolution structures of proteins, nucleic acids, and other biomolecules; (vi) the utilization of powerful spectroscopic tools allowing studies of structures and dynamics; and (vii) more recently, the widespread use of macromolecular engineering to create new biologically relevant structures at will. All this and more is reflected in the volumes of the series *Metal Ions in Life Sciences*.

---

* Reproduced with some alterations by permission of John Wiley & Sons, Ltd., Chichester, UK (copyright 2006) from pages v and vi of Volume 1 of the series *Metal Ions in Life Sciences* (MILS-1).

The importance of metal ions to the vital functions of living organisms, hence, to their health and well-being, is nowadays well accepted. However, in spite of all the progress made, we are still only at the brink of understanding these processes. Therefore, the series Metal Ions in Life Sciences links coordination chemistry and biochemistry in their widest sense. Despite the evident expectation that a great deal of future outstanding discoveries will be made in the interdisciplinary areas of science, there are still "language" barriers between the historically separate spheres of chemistry, biology, medicine, and physics. Thus, it is one of the aims of this series to catalyze mutual "understanding." It is our hope that Metal Ions in Life Sciences continues to prove a stimulus for new activities in the fascinating "field" of Biological Inorganic Chemistry. If so, it will well serve its purpose and be a rewarding result for the efforts spent by the authors.

Astrid Sigel and Helmut Sigel
Department of Chemistry, Inorganic Chemistry
University of Basel, CH-4056 Basel, Switzerland

Eva Freisinger and Roland K. O. Sigel
Department of Chemistry
University of Zürich, CH-8057 Zürich, Switzerland

October 2005 and March 2023

Preface to Volume 26

Metal-Containing Molecules and Nanomaterials:

From Diagnosis to Therapy

I am delighted to have the opportunity to edit a volume for the famed *Metal Ions in Life Sciences* series and contribute to its tradition of highlighting the latest research findings in inorganic chemistry and coordination chemistry relevant to the life sciences. The public is often unaware of the central role of metals and their ions, and it is only in more advanced chemistry classes that students in the sciences learn the central role they play for all living beings. In this volume, we focus on the use of metal ions in compounds and materials for disease diagnosis and therapy.

Arsphenamine, more commonly known as Salvarsan, an arsenic-containing molecule that was used by Paul Ehrlich's laboratory as an alternative to mercury-containing compounds in the treatment of syphilis, and cisplatin and its widespread use as a cancer drug, heralded the era of metallodrugs. Metallodrugs are effective in combating disease through myriad mechanisms; thus, the potential combinations of drugs and diseases are plentiful.

Moreover, metals and metal-containing molecules have properties such as an electrochemical or an optical signal that can be used to diagnose specific biologically relevant molecules or unravel cellular metabolism; therefore, they are of interest in diagnosis as well.

Additionally, metals are part of the elements essential for life, such as iron and its central role in oxygen transport as part of the hemoglobin protein in red blood cells, or cobalamin, more commonly referred to as vitamin B12, that has a cobalt center and is involved in several biological processes, such as DNA synthesis and amino acid metabolism. Cobalamin is a water-soluble vitamin and must be sourced, for humans, from animal-derived food or supplements, and this is the case for many other life-essential metals; thus, metal-containing molecules are receiving increased attention in nutraceuticals.

The authors in this book are preeminent bioinorganic, medicinal inorganic chemists, and electrochemists. In this volume, they review the most current research in their area of expertise, assembling knowledge that can be used by the scientific community to continue increasing the relevance of metal-containing molecules and nanomaterials for diagnosis and therapy and thus increase the practical use of these systems.

The content of this book is suitable for researchers in bioinorganic chemistry, coordination chemistry, physical inorganic chemistry, medicinal chemistry, pharmacy, and drug design and discovery, as well as a reference for graduate students in the same fields.

Ana de Bettencourt-Dias

Contents

Contributors to Volume 26

Elmira Alipour
Department of Physics
Wake Forest University
Winston-Salem, NC 27109, USA

Mario A. Alpuche-Aviles
Department of Chemistry
University of Nevada, Reno
Reno, NV 89557, USA

Amanda Blanque Becceneri
Faculty of Pharmaceutical Sciences of
Ribeirão Preto
Universidade de São Paulo
Ribeirão Preto – SP, Brazil,
14040-903

Mauro Botta
Departimento di Scienze e
Innovazione Tecnologica
Università del Piemonte Orientale
"Amedeo Avogadro"
I-15121 Alessandria, Italy

Debbie C. Crans
Department of Chemistry
Colorado State University
Fort Collins, CO 80523, USA
and
Cell and Molecular Biology Program
Colorado State University
Fort Collins, CO 80523, USA

Madeline Denison
Department of Chemistry
Wayne State University
Detroit, MI 48202, USA

Rebeca L. Fernandez
Department of Chemistry
University of California, Davis
Davis, CA 95616, USA

Peter C. Ford
Department of Chemistry and
Biochemistry
University of California, Santa Barbara
Santa Barbara, CA 93110-9510, USA

Mark T. Gladwin
Department of Medicine
University of Maryland School of
Medicine
Baltimore, MD 21201, USA

Marie C. Heffern
Department of Chemistry
University of California, Davis
Davis, CA 95616, USA

Daniel B. Kim-Shapiro
Department of Physics
Wake Forest University
Winston-Salem, NC 27109, USA

Kameron Klugh
Department of Chemistry
Colorado State University
Fort Collins, CO 80523, USA

Jeremy J. Kodanko
Department of Chemistry
Wayne State University
Detroit, MI 48202, USA
and
Barbara Ann Karmanos Cancer
Institute
Detroit, MI 48201, USA

Kateryna Kostenkova
Department of Chemistry
Colorado State University
Fort Collins, CO 80523, USA

Vanessa J. Lee
Department of Chemistry
University of California, Davis
Davis, CA 95616, USA

Francisco Rinaldi Neto
Faculty of Pharmaceutical Sciences of
Ribeirão Preto
Universidade de São Paulo
Ribeirão Preto – SP, Brazil,
14040-903

Roberto Santana da Silva
Faculty of Pharmaceutical Sciences of
Ribeirão Preto
Universidade de São Paulo
Ribeirão Preto – SP, Brazil,
14040-903
and
Department of Chemistry and
Biochemistry
University of California, Santa
Barbara
Santa Barbara, CA 93110-9510, USA

Matheus Torelli Martin
Faculty of Pharmaceutical Sciences of
Ribeirão Preto
Universidade de São Paulo
Ribeirão Preto – SP, Brazil,
14040-903

Claudia Turro
Department of Chemistry and
Biochemistry
The Ohio State University
Columbus, OH 43210, USA

Mark Woods
Department of Chemistry
Portland State University
Portland, OR 97201, USA
and
Advanced Imaging Research Center
Oregon Health & Science University
Portland, OR 97201, USA

Handbooks and Book Series Published and (Co-)edited by the SIGELs

"Handbook on Toxicity of Inorganic Compounds" (ISBN: 0-8247-7727-1) Eds H. G. Seiler, H. Sigel, A. Sigel; Dekker, Inc.; New York; 1988; 1069 pp

"Handbook on Metals in Clinical and Analytical Chemistry" (ISBN: 0-8247-9094-4) Eds H. G. Seiler, A. Sigel, H. Sigel; Dekker, Inc.; New York, Basel, Hong Kong; 1994; 753 pp

"Handbook on Metalloproteins" (ISBN: 0-8247-0520-3) Eds I. Bertini, A. Sigel, H. Sigel; Marcel Dekker, Inc.; New York, Basel; 2001; 1182 pp

Metal Ions in Biological Systems
Volumes 1–44
https://www.routledge.com/Metal-Ions-in-Biological-Systems/book-series/ IHCMEIOBISY
(see also the website given below)

Metal Ions in Life Sciences
Volumes 1–27
Details about all books (series) edited by the SIGELs, including the Guest Editors, can be found at http://www.bioinorganic-chemistry.org/mils

1 Electrochemical Sensors with Inorganic Redox Mediators

Mario A. Alpuche-Aviles
Department of Chemistry
University of Nevada, Reno
Reno, Nevada 89557, USA
malpuche@unr.edu

CONTENTS

ABSTRACT

This chapter covers sensors based on electrogenerated chemiluminescence (ECL) and glucose sensors based on redox hydrogels. These sensing devices rely on electrochemical reactions and are commercially available while continuing to be the object of research and development. The sensors presented here use redox mediators to bypass the limitations of long-range electron transfer. The chapter includes a theoretical background of redox mediators and presents some fundamental equations for electron transfer kinetics. ECL uses redox mediators to excite an electrochemical tag that is a reporter of an antigen/antibody conjugation and is used in commercially available immunoassays. This chapter also covers some selected

DOI: 10.1201/9781003361756-1

1

references on the theoretical and historical development of the techniques, e.g., references on the $Ru(bpy)_3^{2+}$/tripropylamine system used in commercial ECL devices. The chapter further discusses glucose sensors based on hydrogels that contain redox centers attached to the polymer backbone. These redox centers transfer electrons from a glucose oxidase (GOx) to the electrode surface. The chapter discusses the electron transport rate through the hydrogel, where the flexibility of the tethers that link the redox centers facilitates electron transfer from the electrode surface to the redox center of GOx.

KEYWORDS

Electrochemistry; Electroanalysis; Glucose; Electrochemiluminescence

1   INTRODUCTION

This chapter covers the use of electroactive species, redox mediators, for electrochemical-based sensors. There are many examples of analytical techniques that rely on electrochemistry. However, some applications do not constitute "sensors". Although the term "sensor" can be problematic, as discussed below, this chapter covers specific examples of electrochemical reactions that mediate electron transfer to detect molecules in solution. These rely on redox mediators, that is, electroactive species that cycle through oxidation states to shuttle electrons back and forth. In their simplest form, a redox mediation is given by two chemical species that oxidize and reduce each other. If R_1 is the species being oxidized, then we have reaction (1):

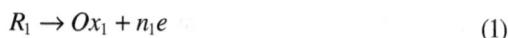

$$R_1 \rightarrow Ox_1 + n_1e \tag{1}$$

where Ox_1 is the product of the oxidation. For the redox mediation to be complete, an oxidizing agent will drive reaction (1), denoted Ox_2:

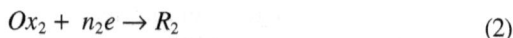

$$Ox_2 + n_2e \rightarrow R_2 \tag{2}$$

So, the overall reaction is:

$$Ox_2 + R_1 \rightarrow Ox_1 + R_2 \tag{3}$$

assuming $n_1 = n_2$.

1.1   THERMODYNAMICS

For the overall reaction (3) to be thermodynamically feasible, the half-reactions (1) and (2) are selected with the primary requirement that $E^{0'2} > E^{0'1}$, where $E^{0'1}$ is the formal potential for the reaction written as a reduction (reverse of reaction (1)), and $E^{0'2}$ is the formal potential of reaction (2), so that $\Delta G_{rxn,3} < 0$, using the usual thermodynamic conventions.

1.2 KINETICS

The rate for the overall reaction (3) follows Marcus theory of electron transfer. In the simplest case, reactions (1) and (2) are outer-sphere, i.e., electron transfer does not involve bond braking, making, or major structural rearrangements. For example, in the reduction of ruthenium(III) hexamine chloride there are only differences in charge between the oxidized and reduced species due to the addition or removal of one electron:

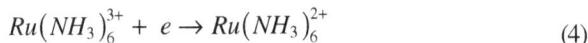

$$Ru(NH_3)_6^{3+} + e \rightarrow Ru(NH_3)_6^{2+} \tag{4}$$

Other examples include ferricyanide $Fe(CN)_6^{3-/4}$, ferrocene, and ferrocene derivatives (e.g., Fc-CH$_3$OH). These outer-sphere redox couples are widely used in electrochemical experiments because the oxidized and reduced species can be stable under certain conditions. In designing redox mediators, one of the species is usually chosen for its stability and, therefore, for the chemical reversibility of the redox process.

The overall reaction (3), the kinetic rate constant, can be described using Marcus theory. Following some of the early nomenclature, the rate constant for the overall reaction between the two redox species in solution is k_{12} [1]:

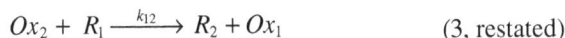

$$Ox_2 + R_1 \xrightarrow{k_{12}} R_2 + Ox_1 \tag{3, restated}$$

The reaction rate, k_{12}, is given by:

$$k_{12} = \sqrt{k_1 k_2 K_{12} f} \tag{5}$$

where k_{11} and k_{22} are rate constants for the electron self-exchange reactions of each half-reaction, and K_{12}=equilibrium constant for the electron transfer reaction (3), which can be calculated with the formal potential, E^0. The parameter f is a constant given by:

$$\log f = \frac{\sqrt{\log K_{12}}}{4 log\left(k_1 k_2 / z^2\right)} \tag{6}$$

where z is the collision frequency of two uncharged molecules in solution; often $z = 10^{11} mol^{-1}/s^{-1}$, and f is close to unity [2].

This reaction scheme is analogous to a redox titration in classical analytical chemistry where one of the species, e.g., R_1, will be the analyte, and the titration will provide a quantitative analysis of R_1. However, in the applications discussed here, mediators enable the detection of analytes at concentrations much smaller than those typically targeted with bulk volumetric titrations. Alternatively, redox mediation can be a way to report on an event, somewhat remote to the electrode surface, such as an antibody (Ab)/antigen (An) binding. Therefore, this chapter covers analytical applications that leverage a redox mediator cycle to achieve the detection of analytes in solution. For example, redox mediators are used for glucose sensing by communicating with a glucose oxidase (GOx) in an application corresponding to one of the highest degrees of development for sensing devices.

1.3 WHAT IS A SENSOR?

Interestingly, to date, there is no official IUPAC definition of a sensor. Paraphrasing the NIST definition to transfer the concepts into a chemical context, a sensor is a device that outputs an electric or optical signal that is readily converted into a concentration [3,4]. Moreover, IUPAC defines biosensors as devices that use biochemical reactions mediated by "enzymes, immune systems, tissues, organelles, or whole cells" to detect a compound [5]. Here, "bio" corresponds to the mechanism of sensing, and in some other contexts, the use of "bio-" will denote the biological function of the molecule of interest. In general, the term sensor refers to a transducing device, i.e., a sensing element that converts a chemical signal into a readily used signal, e.g., electrical or optical. This chapter covers two types of sensors that rely on electrochemical reactions: glucose sensors, which have an electric input and output, and electrogenerated chemiluminescence (ECL) detection, which requires the light emitted to be converted to an electric signal. However, this definition of a sensor as a device corresponds to a higher degree of research and development, such as in commercially available handheld sensors and benchtop instruments. In research, one often chooses to focus on developing a transducing element, as this would be the critical part of the device or a possible future device. Therefore, many articles cover "sensors," but the topic described is often far from a practical device. Instead, many publications cover different stages of developing a chemical transducing element, and many of these published "sensors" require a calibration curve. Accordingly, many journals expand the definition to include sensing mechanisms more generally. Table 1 shows a few of the journals that cover this topic.

TABLE 1

Examples of Journals Dedicated to Publish Significant Contributions to Sensing Mechanisms as of 2023

Journal	Publisher
ACS Sensors	American Chemical Society
Analyst	Royal Society of Chemistry
Analytical Chemistry	American Chemical Society
ECS Sensors Plus	The Electrochemical Society
Frontiers in Sensors	Frontiers
Sensors and Actuators B: Chemical	Elsevier
Sensors and Diagnostics	Royal Society of Chemistry

1.4 CHAPTER SCOPE

There is a vast literature on the applications of sensors for analytical chemistry, with many journals dedicated to the subject (Table 1). For some time now, sensors have been the object of research and development, and therefore, in this chapter, we will not attempt a comprehensive review of chemical sensors. Instead, we will focus on two analytical applications with well-established electrochemical solutions that rely on inorganic materials and redox couples.

Because electrochemical sensors convert chemical quantities into electric signals, there is a wide range of analytes that can be targeted without necessarily building a device but by focusing research efforts on the transducing mechanisms, i.e., the electrochemical process that provides a means to detect a chemical species, without necessarily worrying about the final output signal. This chapter presents glucose sensors as some of the most advanced examples of redox-mediated, enzyme-based electrochemical sensors. We also cover ECL because, like glucose sensors, there are commercially available ECL sensors that rely on this sensing mechanism [6].

1.5 ELISA AND IMMUNOASSAYS

Immunoassays rely on the binding between antibodies (Ab) and antigens (An); however, the Ab/An binding is usually insufficient to perform analysis. Therefore, immunoassays rely on some transducing signal, e.g., a tag that can report on the Ab/An binding. Initially, ELISA designated a very particular kind of immunoassay, namely an enzyme-linked immunosorbent assay [7]. This type of analysis is depicted in Figure 1a. In this type of analysis, the antibody bound to the substrate is exposed to a solution that contains the antigen. After incubation, the antibody bound to the surface is conjugated with the antigen. After washing to remove unbound species, the substrate is exposed to a solution containing an antibody chemically bound to an enzyme. The antigen is then "sandwiched" between antibodies. The substrate is usually rewashed, and the enzyme produces a photoluminescent compound. This type of Ab/An/Ab "sandwich" gives ELISA specificity, as this type of test will be very selective toward an antigen; however, the test can be modified to make the Ab the analytical target. Antibodies can be isolated from biological fluids or produced for a specific antigen, giving ELISA great flexibility. There are different types of inmunoassays and detection arrangements, but the Ab/An bioconjugate remains central to the test's specificity. The enzyme-modified antibody functions as a tag because the enzyme yields products that can be detected by absorbance, fluorescence, or radioactive labeling [8]. Modern immunoassays derive from the pioneering work of Rossalyn Yalow [9], who demonstrated that isotopes could track Ab/An binding. Since then, these methods have been constantly reviewed to improve their sensitivity, such as in time-resolved immunoassays [10]. However, many authors consider ELISA distinct in that it happens in the solid state. In practice, ELISA methods use plastic plates in well formats, and there are many instruments

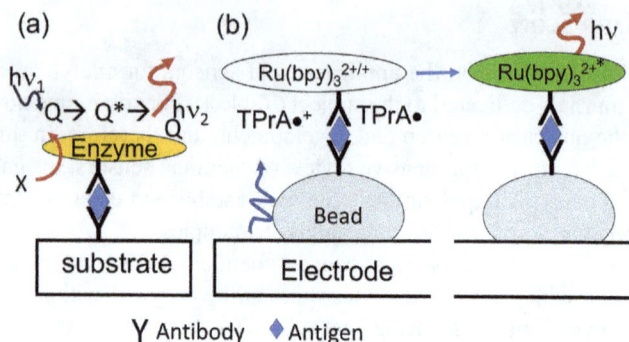

(a)   (b)

Y Antibody   ♦ Antigen

FIGURE 1 (a) Schematic representation of an ELISA test: an enzyme turns over a photoluminescent product, and the fluorescence generates an analytical signal. (b) An ECL-based detection with a similar approach, where $Ru(bpy)_3^{2+}$ is used as the analytical tag in an aqueous solution. The signal comes from the electrochemically generated chemiluminescence; the working electrode oxidizes tri-n-propyl amine (TPrA), and the oxidation products, $TPrA^+$ and $TPrA^+$, generate the excited state $Ru(bpy)_3^{2+*}$ that ultimately emits light.

designed specifically for "reading plates." Besides the availability of specialized equipment, there are other advantages to ELISA methods, among them that it uses small volumes of reactants, is sensitive, and leverages the sensitivity of photoluminescence; it has become a standard in immunoassay and an essential diagnostic tool [9]. Therefore, there has been a drive to implement different sensing mechanisms around the Ab/An binding that have yielded different types of immunoassays.

A similar immunoassay that this chapter includes is ECL. Like chemiluminescence methods, ECL increases the signal-to-noise ratio because they do not require an external excitation source that can introduce background noise when trying to detect the emission from an analyte, as in the case of ELISA [11]. Also, from an instrumentation point of view, there is no need for an external light source. In this type of immunoassay, the ruthenium complex tris(bipyridine) ruthenium(II), $Ru(bpy)_3^{2+}$, is the most widely used emitter in aqueous systems. It is usually employed with a co-reactant. The co-reactant generates an oxidizer and reducing agent, e.g., tri-n-propyl amine (TPrA) produces oxidizing and reducing agents when it is oxidized in aqueous solutions at a pH of around 7. Because of its stability in aqueous conditions, commercial ECL technology employs the TPrA/ $Ru(bpy)_3^{2+}$ couple. To facilitate the application of ECL, the analyzers use magnetic beads decorated with antibodies, and in the last step of the immunoassay, a $Ru(bpy)_3^{2+}$-modified antibody, provides the label. Figure 1b shows a schematic of this configuration. The electrode oxidizes TPrA, and this produces $TPrA^+$ and $TPrA^{*+}$; the mechanism is complex, but the $TPrA^+$ and $TPrA^{*+}$ generate the excited state $Ru(bpy)_3^{2+*}$ which emits the light used for the analysis.

2   ELECTROGENERATED CHEMILUMINESCENCE

In ECL, light results from an excited species that is electrochemically generated; that is, the excited state is formed in a reaction between two species in solution that were generated by electrochemical reactions. This analytical technique is sensitive to picomolar levels, thanks in part to the fact that it does not require a light source and, therefore, has intrinsically lower background levels [12]. The luminescence arises from redox-active species that ultimately generate an excited state. For example, reactants A and D will undergo electrochemical reduction and oxidation at the electrode surface, and their products will react in solution to generate light in a sequence of reactions [12]:

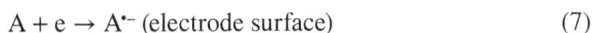

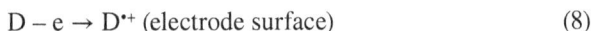

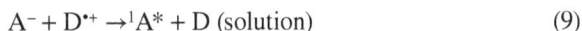

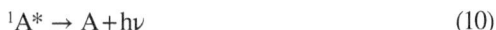

$$A + e \rightarrow A^{\cdot -} \text{ (electrode surface)} \qquad (7)$$

$$D - e \rightarrow D^{\cdot +} \text{ (electrode surface)} \qquad (8)$$

$$A^- + D^{\cdot +} \rightarrow {}^1A^* + D \text{ (solution)} \qquad (9)$$

$${}^1A^* \rightarrow A + h\nu \qquad (10)$$

Reactions (7) and (8) produce radicals that are high-energy species with respect to their parent molecules. In the so-called single systems, the parent molecules are the same in reactions (7) and (8).

2.1   MODEL COMPOUND

In ECL, 9,10-diphenylanthracene (DPA) is a model compound [13]; in an organic solvent (e.g., acetonitrile), the reactions and their electrochemical potentials are [13,14]:

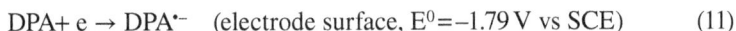

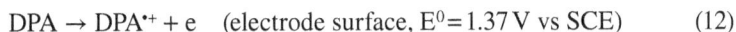

$$DPA + e \rightarrow DPA^{\cdot -} \quad \text{(electrode surface, } E^0 = -1.79 \text{ V vs SCE)} \qquad (11)$$

$$DPA \rightarrow DPA^{\cdot +} + e \quad \text{(electrode surface, } E^0 = 1.37 \text{ V vs SCE)} \qquad (12)$$

In practice, one prepares a solution of DPA and then pulses the potential of an electrode from the positive and negative regions to generate the two radicals in reactions (11) and (12), respectively. The radicals generated at the electrode surface diffuse away from the electrode, and in solution, the radical ions will form an encounter complex [13]:

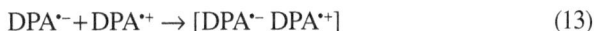

$$DPA^{\cdot -} + DPA^{\cdot +} \rightarrow [DPA^{\cdot -} \; DPA^{\cdot +}] \qquad (13)$$

This complex can result in two neutral molecules via three different reactions [13]:

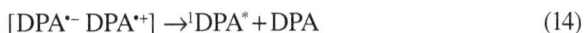

$$[DPA^{\cdot -} \; DPA^{\cdot +}] \rightarrow {}^1DPA^* + DPA \qquad (14)$$

$$[DPA^{\bullet -}\ DPA^{\bullet +}] \rightarrow {}^{3}DPA^{*} + DPA \tag{15}$$

$$[DPA^{\bullet -}\ DPA^{\bullet +}] \rightarrow 2DPA \tag{16}$$

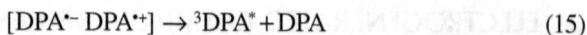

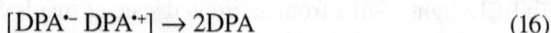

When the radical ions react in solution, their excess energy is large ($\Delta E^{0} = 3.16\,\text{V}$) and can be sufficient to populate the singlet state (14). Reaction (16) will be slow because of the reorganization energy and Marcus's inverted region [11]. The photoluminescence efficiency of DPA is 1 [13]; however, in ECL experiments, the efficiency approaches 25% because the spin-statistics of the annihilating reaction indicate that 25% is the theoretical maximum of the formation of DPA singlets, reaction (14) [15]. The DPA example illustrates the mechanism of ECL emission and showcases some insights that ECL studies can yield. Initially, ECL studies focused on organic molecules, and studies of metal chelates came later, and in time, this evolved into ECL applications in routine analysis.

2.2 RUTHENIUM-BASED LUMINOPHORES

The use of ruthenium-based luminophores has been pivotal to the use of ECL in analysis, including immunoassays [6] and DNA detection [16], in part because $Ru(bpy)_3^{2+}$ and its derivatives can be used as ECL luminophores in aqueous solutions. The photoluminescence of $Ru(bpy)_3^{2+}$ was studied in the 1960s. In 1972, Tokel and Bard demonstrated ECL from the annihilation reactions studied in aprotic media (MeCN) [17]. The reactions and their potentials are [17]:

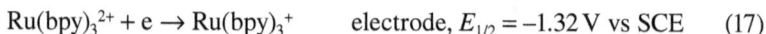

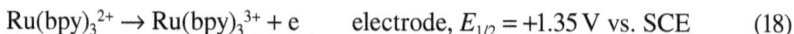

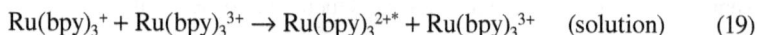

$$Ru(bpy)_3^{2+} + e \rightarrow Ru(bpy)_3^{+} \qquad \text{electrode, } E_{1/2} = -1.32\,\text{V vs SCE} \tag{17}$$

$$Ru(bpy)_3^{2+} \rightarrow Ru(bpy)_3^{3+} + e \qquad \text{electrode, } E_{1/2} = +1.35\,\text{V vs. SCE} \tag{18}$$

$$Ru(bpy)_3^{+} + Ru(bpy)_3^{3+} \rightarrow Ru(bpy)_3^{2+*} + Ru(bpy)_3^{3+} \qquad \text{(solution)} \tag{19}$$

$Ru(bpy)_3^{2+}$ has become the most widely studied ECL molecule because of its application in commercial ECL instruments [18]. However, note that the potentials for reactions (17) and (18) are not accessible in aqueous solutions with most electrode materials available to date. As in the case of DPA, there is a sizeable potential gap between the oxidation and reduction potentials needed to produce the oxidized and reduced species that will, in turn, generate the excited state. One way to circumvent this problem in aqueous solution is to use co-reactants and remove the need for large potential step cycles between the reactions that form the reacting species, e.g., reactions (17) and (18). A co-reactant is a species that, upon oxidation, can generate a reducing agent or an oxidizing agent after being reduced. The most widely used co-reactant for $Ru(bpy)_3^{2+}$ is TPrA. Since it was first reported in 1990 [19], TPrA and $Ru(bpy)_3^{2+}$ allowed the generation of $Ru(bpy)_3^{2+*}$ in aqueous solutions at pH around 7, that is, close to physiological pH, which effectively enabled the use of ECL in immunoassays. Because of the broad applicability of the TPrA – $Ru(bpy)_3^{2+}$ pair, the mechanism to generate the excited

state has been extensively studied [19,20], and it is now considered well understood [21]. Since the reports of the chemiluminescence of the TPrA – $Ru(bpy)_3^{3+}$
[20] and the early reports of the use of TPrA as a co-reactant in ECL [19], the
ECL reaction mechanism was known to include the following reactions when the
electrode is biased to oxidize the reactants, e.g., $E_{app}=0.9$ vs. SCE [22]:

$$Ru(bpy)_3^{2+} \rightarrow Ru(bpy)_3^{3+} + e \text{ (electrode)} \tag{20}$$

$$TPrA \rightarrow TPrA^{\bullet+} + e \quad \text{(electrode)} \tag{21}$$

$$TPrA^{\bullet+} \rightarrow TPrA^{\bullet} + H^+ \tag{22}$$

$$Ru(bpy)_3^{3+} + TPrA^{\bullet} \rightarrow Ru(bpy)_3^{2+*} + P \tag{23}$$

where P represents the final oxidation product, $EtCHNPr_2^+$ [21]. Reactions (20) to
(23) show the chemistry of a co-reactant similar to other co-reactants, e.g., oxa-
late [23]. However, this mechanism did not account for some features of the ECL
experiment, and thus, it was further investigated [21]. Miao et al. [21] proposed a
mechanism that includes, in addition to reactions (20) to (23), a route that involves
the radical cation, $TPrA^+$, reacting with $Ru(bpy)^{3+}$ to generate the excited state:

$$Ru(bpy)^{3+} + TPrA^{\bullet+} \rightarrow Ru(bpy)_3^{2+*} \tag{24}$$

They found that even though the radical cation is relatively short-lived, with a
half-life of ca. 0.2 ms, under the right conditions enough of it can diffuse toward
the $Ru(bpy)^{3+}$ to play a significant role in the generation of the excited state
$Ru(bpy)_3^{2+*}$. The overall mechanism is complicated, as can be seen in Figure 2,
which only includes the contribution of the radical cation. The authors proposed
the radical cation as a significant contributor to ECL based on experiments that
included electron paramagnetic resonance (EPR) coupled with electrochemistry.

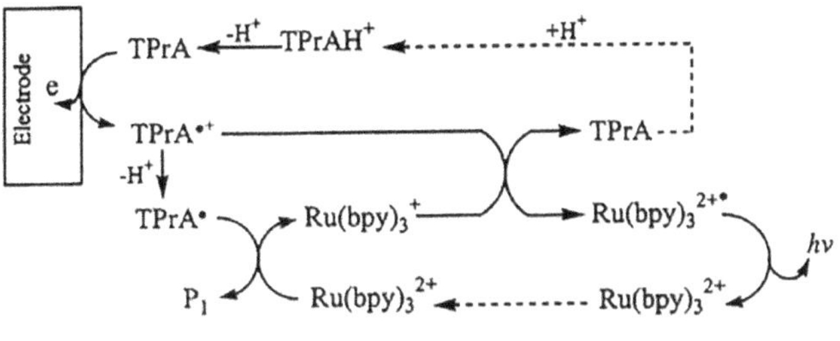

FIGURE 2 Simplified mechanism of the excitation of $Ru(bby)_3^{2+}$ with TPrA; this is an
additional route that generates the excited state $Ru(bby)_3^{2+*}$. (Reprinted with permission
from Ref. [21]. Copyright 2002, American Chemical Society).

Overall, in the aqueous ECL generation with the TPrA – Ru(bpy)$_3^{2+}$ pair, three reactions generate the excited state, Ru(bpy)$_3^{2+*}$:

  i. The annihilation of Ru(bpy)$_3^{3+}$ and Ru(bpy)$_3^{+}$, reaction (19), although the Ru(bpy)$_3^{+}$ species is generated by the co-reactant in the proximity of the electrode surface (Figure 2);
 ii. Reaction of TPrA and Ru(bpy)$_3^{3+}$, reaction (23); and
iii. Reaction of Ru(bpy)$^{3+}$ and TPrA^{+}, reaction (24).

While the mechanism was not well understood until 2002, the fact that Ru(bpy)$_3^{2+*}$ is the excited state has long been accepted based on the ECL spectra. Figure 3 shows an example of the spectra generated during ECL using a glassy carbon electrode in a buffer system at pH 7.5.

   Miao and Choi point out that the complex mechanism illustrates the challenging design of a co-reactant for aqueous solutions [24]. The redox potentials of the TPrA$^{•}$ and TPrA$^{•+}$ species must be adequate to reduce and oxidize the Ru(bpy)$_3^{2+}$ label. The lifetime of the short-lived species must allow for sufficient concentrations of the redox mediators to build up in the proximity of the electrode to generate the excited state. In addition to these challenges, the ECL efficiency of Ru(bpy)$_3^{2+/3+}$ in MeCN is ca. 5% [25,26], while its photoluminescence efficiency is ca. 6% [27]. Therefore, many metal chelate systems have been proposed [18] because it is desirable to have a higher-efficiency ECL system, resulting in higher sensitivity for analytical applications. Also, alternative co-reactant systems suitable for aqueous work could allow the use of different potential windows, electrode materials, or emission wavelengths [18,24].

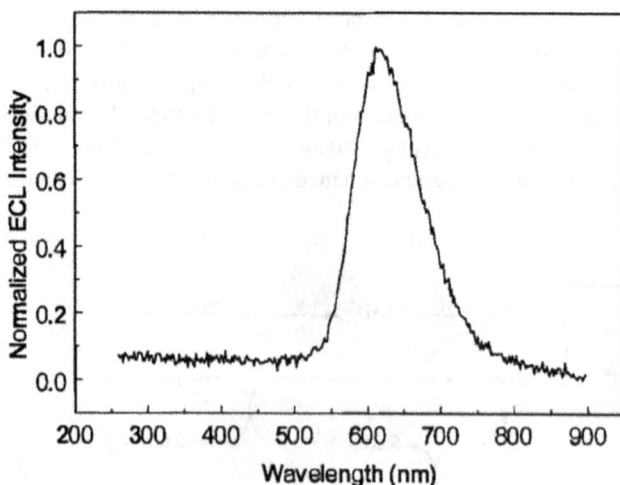

FIGURE 3 ECL normalized spectrum from 1 μM Ru(bpy)$_3^{2+}$ and 100 mM TPrA. The spectrum was generated with a glassy carbon electrode, $E = 0.9$ V vs. SCE, in buffer (0.15 M phosphate, pH 7.5). (Reprinted with permission from Ref. [22]. Copyright 2000, American Chemical Society).

3 GLUCOSE SENSORS

3.1 OVERVIEW

Glucose sensors are among the most developed electrochemical devices and have evolved into "point-of-care" devices, i.e., the patient can use these sensors without any input from a facility or a medical professional. The type of sensing mechanism described here is part of a self-standing device that can provide glucose concentration measurements at short intervals, e.g., every minute [28], therefore approaching "real time." The requirements for accuracy for these types of sensors are critical because, literally, for many patients, the use of insulin depends on the reading on the device. The challenges of glucose monitoring include that glucose concentration levels vary during the day. Therefore, the sensor needs to have a dynamic range that covers the concentration ranges for non-diabetic individuals (4–8 mM) and diabetic patients (2–30 mM) [29]. The glucose concentration can also change through different body parts, and many commercial sensors require blood from the fingertips; e.g., blood from the forearm may have different concentrations than from the fingertips [30]. Many devices require the patient to draw blood and then provide a small drop on the strip with the electrodes printed. However, finger pricking makes some patients fall out of treatment compliance because of the discomfort of continuously pricking the same regions, and some patients skip their glucose tests, which can have long-term health consequences [29,31]. This chapter presents an overview of glucose sensors that rely on enzymes that provide steady-state specificity toward the analyte. The sensing approach relies on subcutaneous glucose detection, removing the need to collect blood samples.

3.2 SOME CHALLENGES WITH ENZYME-BASED ELECTRODES

One issue that makes the immobilization of enzymes on electrodes challenging when using enzymes in electrochemical detection is that enzymes may be denatured when immobilized onto electrode surfaces. Denaturalization happens when, upon immobilizing the enzyme, the tertiary native structure is lost, resulting in a different arrangement of the polypeptide chain because the electrode environment (e.g., a metal) can distort the electrostatic interactions that stabilize the structure, deteriorating enzymatic activity [32,33]. Therefore, the enzyme is usually supported away from the electroactive area, as depicted in Figure 4a. In what is considered [34] the earliest report of a sensor based on GOx immobilization combined with electrochemical measurements, Clark and Lyons [35] immobilized the enzyme on membranes. Later, Updike and Hiss [36] used an acrylamide gel in their 'enzyme electrode.' Hydrogels are now used to modify electrode surfaces to support and stabilize the enzyme and provide electron-conductive paths.

Another problem with using enzymes in electrochemistry is that immobilizing pure enzymes on an electrode surface often does not allow electronic communication between the enzyme redox center and the electrode. Heller [28] notes that many enzymes are too large to allow efficient connection between the electrode and the enzyme redox center. Enzymes have outer shells that usually bury the redox-active center far from the electrode surface. To connect an electrode with an enzyme, electron tunneling will be the primary mechanism to move electrons from the electrode surface to the redox center, and according to theory, the rate of tunneling, k_{et}, is [28,37]:

$$k_{et} = 10^{13} \exp\left[-\beta(d-3)\right]\exp-\frac{\left(\Delta G + \lambda\right)^2}{4RT\lambda} \tag{25}$$

where d is the distance between the donor/acceptor pair, β is a constant for the medium containing the donor/acceptor pair, $-\Delta G$ is the driving energy (e.g., $\Delta G = -e\Delta E^0$), λ is the Marcus reorganization energy, R is the ideal gas constant, and T is the absolute temperature. Because of the $\exp\left[-\beta(d-3)\right]$ factor in Equation 25, longer distances make tunneling inefficient, although direct connection to an enzyme has been achieved [38,39] using a polyvinyl chloride support mixed with conductive organic salts. An alternative approach that has been developed is using redox mediators connected with flexible tethers to relay electrons to and from the enzymatic redox-active site, which allows for connecting the enzymes with the electrode surface and continuous glucose oxidation [40]. The redox center on GOx is flavin adenine dinucleotide (FAD), which cycles between its oxidized (FAD) and reduced forms (FADH$_2$) [29].

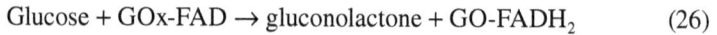

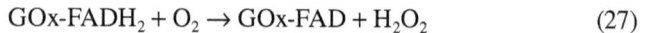

$$\text{Glucose + GOx-FAD} \rightarrow \text{gluconolactone + GO-FADH}_2 \tag{26}$$

$$\text{GOx-FADH}_2 + O_2 \rightarrow \text{GOx-FAD} + H_2O_2 \tag{27}$$

The half-reaction for the redox center is:

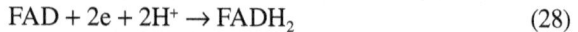

$$\text{FAD} + 2e + 2H^+ \rightarrow \text{FADH}_2 \tag{28}$$

Therefore, a redox mediator will ensure that the FAD regenerates from the reduced form (FADH$_2$) [28,40]. Methylene blue, ferrocene derivatives, and other redox mediators have been tested, and $Fe(CN)_6^{3-/4-}$ is used in some commercial glucose detection strips [29]. The mediators can be in solution, but they must be able to reach the FAD center in the enzyme. Figure 5 shows a schematic representation of how the redox mediators, Ox and Red, can reach the FAD redox center, and these mediators shuttle electrons back to the electrode.

The development of these sensors started in the 1960s. Clark and Lyons [35] immobilized the enzyme on membranes; in this earlier report, they proposed two approaches: (1) using a Cuprophane/GOx/Cuprophane sandwich and a pH electrode to monitor the changes in pH due to the ultimate production of gluconic acid (Figure 4a). (2) Using a polyethylene membrane/dialysis membrane/GOx assembly on an O_2 concentration electrode, they could measure glucose concentration because GOx consumes O_2 as it oxidizes glucose (Figure 4a). This competitive sensing mechanism was later used in the "enzyme electrode" [36], as described

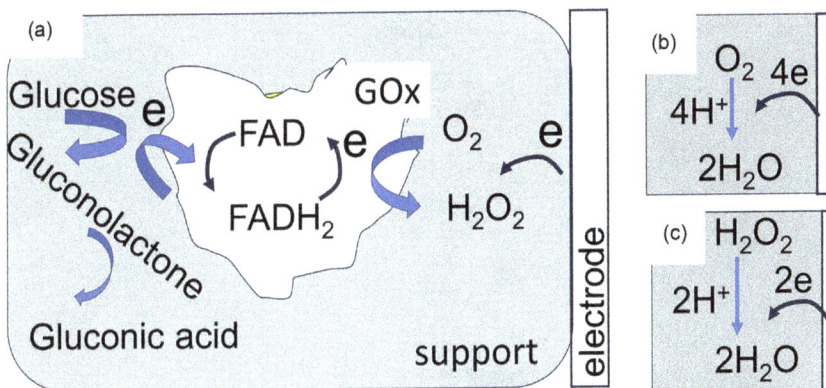

FIGURE 4 (a) Schematic of an electrode modified with GOx. In the 'enzyme electrode,' the enzyme is immobilized with a hydrogel. (b) The electrode reducing O_2 in the gel to provide a competitive detection scheme for the concentration of glucose on the enzyme electrode (reported in Ref. [36]). (c) The detail of the detection scheme where the H_2O_2, produced by the enzyme, is reduced to produce a signal for the glucose concentration.

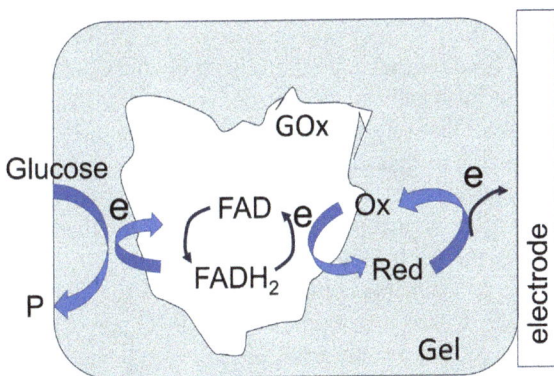

FIGURE 5 Schematic representation of an enzyme-based glucose sensor. The GOx enzyme is immobilized in a gel, and redox mediators Ox and Red shuttle electrons to enable glucose oxidation while cycling FAD from its oxidized to its reduced state $FADH_2$.

above, where reducing the dissolved O_2 provides a measurement of glucose concentration (Figure 4b). In another type of measurement, the electrolysis of H_2O_2 provides the signal because the GOx produces H_2O_2, reaction (27); measuring the peroxide generated can be used to measure glucose concentration. Guilbault and Lubrano [41] used the oxidation of H_2O_2 on a Pt electrode. At pH ca. 7, the potential required to oxidize H_2O_2 is considerably positive, e.g., 0.6 V vs. SCE [41], but potentials in the range of 0.3–0.8 V have been reported [29]. Another approach is reducing H_2O_2 at potentials around −0.1 V vs. SCE, as depicted in Figure 4c. These peroxide-electrolysis schemes are widely used in the scientific

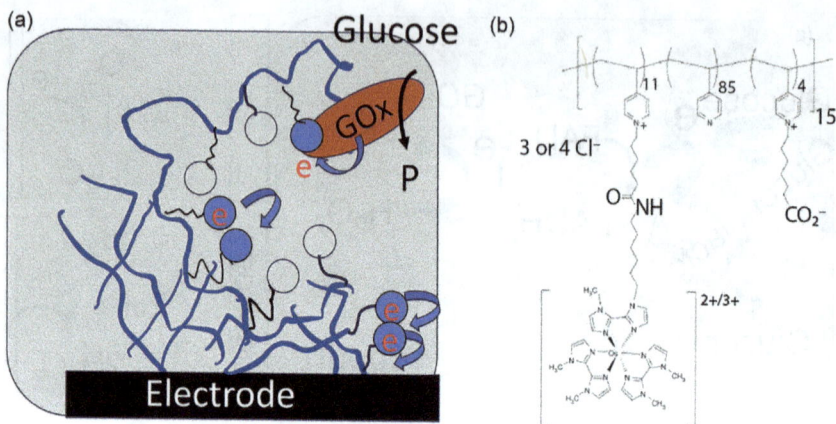

FIGURE 6 (a) Schematic representation of a redox-active hydrogel allowing connection from the electrode to the glucose oxidase enzyme (GOx); the circles represent redox centers that can be Os-based chelates. (b) Redox polymer based on a poly(4-vinylpyridine) backbone modified with an Os-bipyridine derivative using a 13-atom linker from the polymer backbone to the redox center. The polymer was prepared to wire GOx (structure reprinted with permission from Ref. [28]. Copyright 2006, Elsevier).

literature, perhaps because they are relatively straightforward to implement with metal electrodes or, alternatively, with a peroxidase [29]. However, this chapter focuses on sensors that rely on electroactive gels and use the current carried by the redox mediator to measure glucose concentration [28,42,43]. As in the examples above, the enzyme is immobilized on a gel, but in the electroactive gel, the redox mediator is attached to the polymeric backbone of the hydrogel. After cross-linking, the gel is attached to the electrode; in this type of modified electrode there are no leachable components, which is advantageous for *in vivo* measurements [43]. Figure 6a is a schematic of this approach: the gel requires water to allow the redox-active branches of the gel to come into proximity with one another. Electrons transfer from the reduced to the oxidized redox centers, allowing electrons to 'move' or diffuse through the polymeric film and to transfer electrons from the redox center of Gox, to effectively connect the enzyme to the electrode [28,43,44].

3.3 HYDROGEL CONDUCTIVITY

Figure 6b shows the structure of a hydrogel designed for 'wiring' GOx. In this example [45], a relatively long tether of 13 atoms is used as a linker to the redox center because longer linkers facilitate the redox center to balance the negative charge more readily. While the apparent electron diffusion coefficient is a function of other parameters [28,43,44], the fact that increasing the linker length facilitates electron transport is characteristic of the mechanism of hydrogel conductivity, where flexible tethers to the redox centers improve transport [46].

Because electrons diffuse through the hydrogel, Aoki et al. [44] found that the main parameter that determined the apparent diffusion coefficient of electrons, D_{app}, was the flexibility of the polymer backbone branches. With the Os directly attached to the N of the pyridine ring on the polymer backbone, the authors reported a D_{app} of electron diffusion of 3.9×10^{-8} cm^2 s^{-1}. Increasing the number of atoms to 8 in the Os-bpy-N link and, thus, making a longer tether, increased the D_{app} to 7.6×10^{-7} cm^2 s^{-1} [47]. Mao et al. [45] found that increasing the number of atoms in the linker to 18 increases the D_{app} to 5.8×10^{-6} cm^2 s^{-1}; also, the authors found that increasing the linker length facilitates electron transfer to the enzyme NADH$_2$ redox center. In contrast, tunneling across alkyl thiols decreases rapidly with distance because of the exponential dependence on distance d. The tunneling rate, k_{et}, decays proportionally to exp$(-d)$, similarly to the exponential decay in Equation 25, making tunneling across a distance of 13 atoms much less probable than at a single Os-N bond distance (e.g., Ref. [48] and references therein). Heller attributes [28] the higher D_{app}, corresponding to more flexible linkers, to the ability of the redox centers to balance charge. Ions from the solution have to move to counter the negative charge as electrons transfer from the reduced to the oxidized center [46]. This shielding of the counter ions is the limiting step in the electron transfer across the hydrogel [49], so longer, more flexible linkers allow the D_{app} to approach the limiting diffusion coefficient of the counter ion in solution [28].

In addition to the need for gel conductivity, the redox mediator is chosen for its potential to drive the redox enzyme GOx. By changing the metal center or the substituents around the bipyridine, the potential of the polymer can be controlled. Therefore, it is possible to tune the driving for electron transfer (ΔG in Equation 25). For GOx, the mediator must be able to oxidize FADH$_2$ so that it drives glucose oxidation [28,43].

This paper closes with a final note on how these glucose sensors eliminated the requirement of removing blood sampling for glucose measurement. Once the redox system had been optimized, the electrode configuration was prepared on a microscopic scale that could be placed into the skin [31]. Also, the sensor is based on coulometry, which removes the calibration requirement [31]. This is possible because there is a correlation between the blood glucose concentration and the glucose concentration measured subcutaneously on the arm [50,51]. This allows the sensor to be worn as a patch; therefore, this is an example of a 'wearable sensor.' Another consequence of the fact that the needle-type electrode senses glucose concentration subcutaneously when a patient does not have medical impediments to rely on it, is that it does not require the conventional sample acquisition and manipulation (pretreatment, separations, etc.) that have been part of traditional analytical techniques. These sensors provide accurate *in vivo* measurements with the straightforward operation required to deploy them as point-of-care devices. These sensors resulted from early electron transfer studies between electrodes, enzymes, redox mediators, and conductive hydrogels. This approach to connecting to a GOx has been extended to other redox enzymes, and different enzymes and redox centers will need new polymers and redox centers based on the principles described above.

ACKNOWLEDGMENT

This material is based on work supported by the National Science Foundation under Grant No. 2108462.

ABBREVIATIONS AND DEFINITIONS

Ab	antibody
An	antigen
ΔE^0	difference in formal potentials for two reactions
ΔG	free energy change
ΔG_{rxn}	reaction free energy
D_{app}	apparent diffusion coefficient for electrons in a conductive hydrogel
$E^{0'}$	formal potential
E_{app}	applied potential to a working electrode
e	electron
Fc	ferrocene
k_{12}	rate constant for redox exchange
K_{12}	redox reaction equilibrium constant
n	number of electrons: Ox + ne → R
Ox	oxidized form of Ox + e → R
R	gas constant
R	reduced form of Ox + e → R
T	absolute temperature in K
bpy	2,2'-bipyridine
DPA	9,10-diphenyl anthracene
ECL	electrogenerated chemiluminescence
ELISA	enzyme-linked immunosorbent assay
FAD	flavin adenine dinucleotide
GOx	glucose oxidase
IUPAC	International Union of Pure and Applied Chemistry
MeCN	acetonitrile
NIST	National Institute of Standards and Technology
SCE	standard calomel electrode
TPrA	tri-n-propyl amine

REFERENCES

1. R. A. Marcus, *J. Chem. Phys.* **1956**, *24*, 966–978.
2. R. A. Marcus, N. Sutin, *Biochim. Biophys. Acta - Bioenerg.* **1985**, *811*, 265–322.
3. L. Kang, 17th IEEE Instrumentation and Measurement Technology Conference Proceedings, Baltimore, MD.
4. National Institute of Standards and Technology, **2009**. Department of Commerce, Washington DC, Definitions, Updated 2021, https://www.nist.gov/el/intelligent-systems-division-73500/definitions

5. International Union of Pure and Applied Chemistry. "Biosensor' in *IUPAC Compendium of Chemical Terminology*, 3rd ed. International Union of Pure and Applied Chemistry; 2006. Online version 3.0.1, 2019. https://doi.org/10.1351/goldbook. B00663.

6. D. R. Deaver, *Nature* **1995**, *377*, 758–760.

7. E. Engvall, P. Perlmann, *Immunochemistry* **1971**, *8*, 871–874.

8. M. F. Clark, R. M. Lister, M. Bar-Joseph, in *Methods in Enzymology*, Eds. A. Weissbach, H. Weissbach, Academic Press, **1986**, vol. 118, pp. 742–766.

9. R. S. Yalow, *J. Chem. Educ.* **1999**, *76*, 767.

10. E. Reichstein, Y. Shami, M. Ramjeesingh, E. P. Diamandis, *Anal. Chem.* **1988**, *60*, 1069–1074.

11. A. J. Bard, L. R. Faulkner, H. S. White, *Electrochemical Methods: Fundamentals and Applications*, 3rd ed., John Wiley & Sons, New York, 2022.

12. A. J. Bard, in *Electrogenerated Chemiluminescence*, Ed. A. J. Bard, Marcel Dekker, Inc., CRC Press, Boca Raton, **2004**, pp. 273–299.

13. S. P. Forry, R. M. Wightman, in *Electrogenerated Chemiluminescence*, Ed., A. J. Bard, CRC Press, Boca Raton, **2004**, pp. 273–299.

14. F. E. Beideman, D. M. Hercules, *J. Phys. Chem.* **1979**, *83*, 2203–2209.

15. K. M. Maness, R. M. Wightman, *J. Electroanal. Chem.* **1995**, *396*, 85–95.

16. G. F. Blackburn, H. P. Shah, J. H. Kenten, J. Leland, R. A. Kamin, J. Link, J. Peterman, M. J. Powell, A. Shah, D. B. Talley, *Clin. Chem.* **1991**, *37*, 1534–1539.

17. N. E. Tokel, A. J. Bard, *J. Am. Chem. Soc.* **1972**, *94*, 2862–2863.

18. M. M. Richter, in *Electrogenerated Chemiluminescence*, Ed., A. J. Bard, CRC Press, Boca Raton, **2004**, pp. 301–358.

19. J. K. Leland, M. J. Powell, *J. Electrochem. Soc.* **1990**, *137*, 3127.

20. J. B. Noffsinger, N. D. Danielson, *Anal. Chem.* **1987**, *59*, 865–868.

21. W. Miao, J.-P. Choi, A. J. Bard, *J. Am. Chem. Soc.* **2002**, *124*, 14478–14485.

22. Y. Zu, A. J. Bard, *Anal. Chem.* **2000**, *72*, 3223–3232.

23. I. Rubinstein, A. J. Bard, *J. Am. Chem. Soc.* **1981**, *103*, 512–516.

24. W. Miao, J.-P. Choi, in Electrogenerated Chemiluminescence, Ed., A. J. Bard, Ed., CRC Press, Boca Raton, **2004**, pp. 213–272.

25. W. L. Wallace, A. J. Bard, *J. Phys. Chem.* **1979**, *83*, 1350–1357.

26. R. S. Glass, L. R. Faulkner, *J. Phys. Chem.* **1981**, *85*, 1160–1165.

27. J. V. Caspar, T. J. Meyer, *J. Am. Chem. Soc.* **1983**, *105*, 5583–5590.

28. A. Heller, *Curr. Opin. Chem. Biol.* **2006**, *10*, 664–672.

29. A. Heller, B. Feldman, *Chem. Rev.* **2008**, *108*, 2482–2505.

30. K. Jungheim, T. Koschinsky, G. McGarraugh, *Diabetes Care* **2001**, *24*, 1303–1306.

31. A. Heller, E. J. Cairns, *Annu. Rev. Chem. Biomol. Eng.* **2015**, *6*, 1–12.

32. C. Beaufils, H.-M. Man, A. de Poulpiquet, I. Mazurenko, E. Lojou, *Catalysts* 2021, *11*.

33. P. V. Iyer, L. Ananthanarayan, *Process Biochem.* **2008**, *43*, 1019–1032.

34. D. Bruen, C. Delaney, L. Florea, D. Diamond, *Sensors* **2017**, *17*, 1866.

35. L. C. Clark Jr., C. Lyons, *Ann. N. Y. Acad. Sci.* **1962**, *102*, 29–45.

36. S. J. Updike, G. P. Hicks, *Nature* **1967**, *214*, 986–988.

37. D. DeVault, Quantum-Mechanical Tunnelling in Biological Systems, 2nd ed., Cambridge University Press, New York, **1984**.

38. W. J. Albery, P. N. Bartlett, A. E. G. Cass, R. Eisenthal, I. J. Higgins, M. Akhtar, C. R. Lowe, I. J. Higgins, *Philos. Trans. R. Soc. London B: Biol. Sci.* **1987**, *316*, 107–119.

39. W. J. Albery, P. N. Bartlett, D. H. Craston, *J. Electroanal. Chem. Interf. Electrochem.* **1985**, *194*, 223–235.

40. C. Bourdillon, C. Demaille, J. Moiroux, J. M. Saveant, *J. Am. Chem. Soc.* 1993, *115*, 1–10.
41. G. G. Guilbault, G. J. Lubrano, *Anal. Chim. Acta* **1973**, *64*, 439–455.
42. B. A. Gregg, A. Heller, *Anal. Chem.* **1990**, *62*, 258–263.
43. A. Heller, *Acc. Chem. Res.* **1990**, *23*, 128–134.
44. A. Aoki, R. Rajagopalan, A. Heller, *J. Phys. Chem.* **1995**, *99*, 5102–5110.
45. F. Mao, N. Mano, A. Heller, *J. Am. Chem. Soc.* **2003**, *125*, 4951–4957.
46. C. P. Andrieux, J. M. Saveant, *J. Phys. Chem.* **1988**, *92*, 6761–6767.
47. V. Soukharev, N. Mano, A. Heller, *J. Am. Chem. Soc.* **2004**, *126*, 8368–8369.
48. A. Kiani, M. A. Alpuche-Aviles, P. K. Eggers, M. Jones, J. J. Gooding, M. N. Paddon-Row, A. J. Bard, *Langmuir* **2008**, *24*, 2841–2849.
49. N. A. Surridge, C. S. Sosnoff, R. Schmehl, J. S. Facci, R. W. Murray, *J. Phys. Chem.* **1994**, *98*, 917–923.
50. U. Hoss, E. S. Budiman, H. Liu, M. P. Christiansen, *J. Diabetes Sci. Technol.* **2014**, *8*, 89–94.
51. E. Cengiz, W. V. Tamborlane, *Diabetes Technol. Ther.* **2009**, *11*, S-11–S-16.

2 Recent Advances of Medicinal Properties of Vanadium Compounds

Cancer and Other Diseases

Kateryna Kostenkova and Kameron Klugh
Department of Chemistry
Colorado State University
Fort Collins, Colorado, USA

Debbie C. Crans[*]
Department of Chemistry
Colorado State University
Fort Collins, Colorado, USA
Cell and Molecular Biology Program
Colorado State University
Fort Collins, Colorado, USA
Debbie.Crans@colostate.edu

CONTENTS

---

[*] Corresponding author.

DOI: 10.1201/9781003361756-2

ABSTRACT

Vanadium is a non-essential first-row transition metal with reported antidiabetic, anticancer, antiparasitic, and antituberculosis properties. In the last decade,
vanadium(IV/V) coordination complexes, vanadium salts, and polyoxidovanadates have gained attention for anticancer applications due to their ability to affect
signaling pathways, inhibit protein tyrosine phosphatases (PTPs), induce reactive
oxygen species (ROS) formation and lipid peroxidation, and affect metabolism.
Studies have demonstrated a general approach for the development of specific
inhibitors for PTP and their activity *in vitro* and *in vivo*. Herein, we have reviewed
the advanced vanadium anticancer research and related topics over the last 5 years
and put this work in context with previous reports. Recent reports have shown
that vanadium anticancer complexes are structurally diverse with the increase of
novel oxovanadium(IV/V) and dioxovanadium(IV/V) Schiff base complexes for
the treatment of different types of cancer. Oxovanadium(IV) complexes have been
investigated for photodynamic therapy applications and have shown cytotoxicity
in several cancer cell lines. Dioxovanadium(V) dipicolinate complexes and simple
salts are reported to enhance oncolytic viruses for immunotherapy. Vanadium
complexes have also been reported for their antidiabetic and cardiovascular applications, as well as their ability to enhance and inhibit ROS formation and oxidative
stress. Future development of vanadium-based therapeutics would benefit from
considering methods to lower toxicity, increase stability and solubility, enhance
biodistribution, and develop delivery formulations in early stages of the project.

KEYWORDS

Vanadium; Vanadate; Vanadyl Sulfate; Anticancer Agents; Vanadium
Coordination Complexes; Lipid Nanoparticles; Intratumoral Injections;
Reactive Oxygen Species

1   INTRODUCTION: VANADIUM COMPOUNDS IN MEDICINE

Vanadium is a non-essential first-row transition metal that has been underex-
plored for medicinal applications [1–6]. Five of the first-row transition metals –
manganese, iron, cobalt, copper, and zinc – are essential to human health [1].

Three of the non-essential first-row transition metals – chromium, vanadium, and nickel – have beneficial biological effects for the treatment of disease. Chromium, vanadium, and nickel complexes have been investigated in clinical trials, and vanadium is the only non-essential element to exhibit both anticancer and anti-diabetic properties [1,7]. Vanadium and zinc are the two transition metals with the highest natural abundance in the Earth crust (0.008% and 0.019%) and with many biological effects, yet zinc is an essential element but vanadium is not [1,8]. Therefore, the biological and medicinal properties of vanadium compounds have been extensively reviewed [1–3,9]. Vanadium compounds have entered 18 clinical trials as of May 2023, compared to, for example, 2,260 clinical trials with zinc, which have also been extensively reviewed [10–12]. Previous studies with vanadium have investigated the antidiabetic properties of vanadium compounds [7,13–16]. More recently, the anticancer properties of vanadium compounds have gained momentum in the bioinorganic chemistry and medicinal communities, mostly over the last 5–10 years [1,5,9,17–20].

A Web of Science search in May 2023 has shown a significant increase of publications of vanadium compounds in medicine over the last two decades (Figure 1a). We have compared the number of publications mentioning vanadium in cancer and vanadium in diabetes. The findings show that both areas are a smaller sub-area within vanadium in medicine, although vanadium has gained attention for its anticancer applications over the last two decades. Reports of applications of vanadium complexes as antidiabetic agents in Web of Science would be expected to decrease when bis(maltolato)oxovanadium(IV) (BMOV) failed clinical trials and went off patent on September 30, 2011 [7,14,21]. As shown in Figure 1, publications on antidiabetic agents have decreased

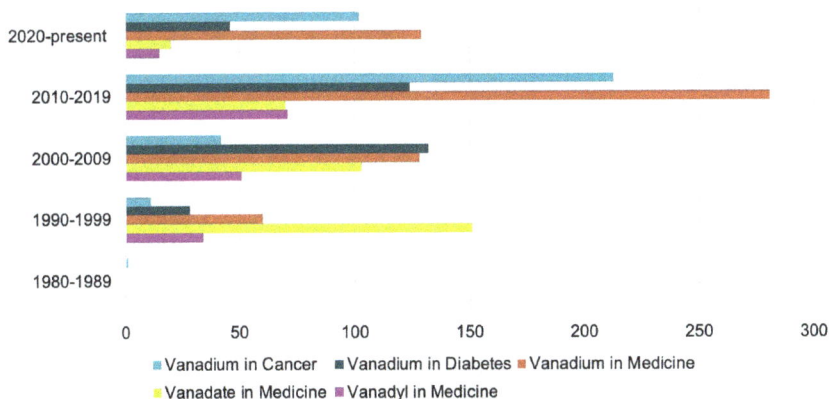

FIGURE 1 Number of reported studies, between 1980 and the present, using vanadyl, vanadate, and vanadium complexes in medicine, cancer, and diabetes. Studies were found by searching the phrases "vanadyl complexes in medicine," "vanadate complexes in medicine," and "vanadium complexes in medicine" on Web of Science.

since 2011. The interest in vanadium has then increased for cancer studies, its involvement in oxidative stress, and emerging diseases such as neurological diseases and SARS [17,22]. Between 2018 and 2023, 269 peer-reviewed publications using vanadium as an anticancer agent have been published. We anticipate that the number of publications involving vanadium in medicine and various diseases will continue to increase in the next 5 years.

As a transition metal ion, vanadium can be a countercation that neutralizes negatively charged residues on biomolecules [23]. Although these systems generally involve vanadium in lower oxidation states, a few systems involve vanadium in oxidation state V, such as the *cis*-dioxovanadium cation. The most frequently observed cases are interactions with proteins, organelles, and involvement in oxidative stress. Interaction of vanadium with transferrin [24] and other blood proteins has been extensively studied. Other enzymes have been reported to bind vanadium in place of its divalent countercation, and some structural details are emerging [25,26]. The effects of vanadium on oxidative stress, lipid peroxidation, and reactive oxygen species (ROS) also involve cationic vanadium species [17]. These modes of action involve Fenton and Haber-Weiss chemistries and various radical species [27,28]. Since vanadium forms many different species under physiological conditions depending on the oxidation state, pH, and metabolites present, the mode of action depends on the species present.

Vanadium in oxidation state five is in the form of vanadate ($H_2VO_4^-$, HVO_4^{2-}) which is a structural and electronic analog of phosphate [25,26]. This form of vanadium can act as a substrate or an inhibitor by interacting with numerous phosphorylase enzymes, including various phosphatases and ribonucleases. The observed inhibition results from the ability of vanadate to bind to the active sites of those enzymes [3,21,29,30]. The inhibition of protein tyrosine phosphatases (PTPs) is responsible for the effects of vanadium on signaling pathways [21]. Physiological effects of vanadium are also caused by the inhibition of the Na^+ and K^+ ATPases; physiological roles include stimulating bone cell proliferation, bone collagen synthesis, neoplastic transformations, and other antidiabetic actions [3]. PTPs have a conservative Cys-His diad in their active site, just like the main protease M^{PRO} in SARS-CoV [22,31]. The reported *in silico* modeling of 20 vanadium complexes in the active site of M^{PR} extends the use of vanadium complexes to the treatment of SARS-CoV2-19 [22].

Several signaling pathways are affected by vanadium compounds, including protein tyrosine kinase receptors [32,33] and G-protein–coupled receptors [34–36], of which the effects on the luteinizing hormone receptor (LHR) have been studied most extensively [36,37]. Recently, it was demonstrated that signaling is sensitive to interaction with the lipid interface [36,37]. Vanadium compounds can activate and deactivate different signaling pathways, and this is important to their antitumoral action [38]. Several signaling pathways activated by vanadium compounds have been identified and include the mitogen-activated protein kinase (MAPK)/extracellular signal-regulated kinase (ERK) signaling pathway, phosphatidylinositol 3-kinase (PI3K)/protein kinase B (AKT) signaling pathways, caspase signaling pathway,

Janus kinase protein (JAK)/signal transducer and activator of transcription protein (STAT) signaling pathway, and nuclear factor erythroid 2–related factor 2 (Nrf2)/ heme oxygenase-1 (HO-1) signaling pathway. Signaling pathways that are inactivated include the focal adhesion kinase (FAK) signaling pathway, autophagy signaling pathway, transforming growth factor beta (TGFbeta)-epithelial-to-mesenchymal transition (EMT) signaling pathway, and Notch-1-signaling pathway. These pathways potentially lead to cell cycle arrest, ROS production, and apoptosis, and the presence of vanadium induces tumor suppressor effects.

One challenge of using vanadium compounds for medicinal applications is the complex vanadium speciation chemistry under physiological conditions [39,40]. Vanadium(V) complexes tend to hydrolyze into vanadate ($H_2VO_4^-$) and a free ligand at physiological pH. Vanadate forms several colorless oxidovanadates with nuclearity of one (V_1, monomer), two (V_2, dimer), four (V_4, tetramer), or five (V_5, pentamer) vanadium atoms, which rapidly interconvert in aqueous solution but can be observed by ^{51}V NMR spectroscopy [40]. The oxidovanadates can, furthermore, have multiple protonation states depending on the pH. Vanadate can also form a polyoxidoanion composed of ten vanadium atoms to make up decavanadate ($V_{10}O_{28}^{6-}$, abbreviated V_{10}) which is stable from pH 3–6.5 [41]. The vanadium speciation chemistry under cellular conditions forms other coordination complexes and oxidovanadates, and it is difficult to know what the active species is [30]. Several oxidovanadates have been reported to have antidiabetic [42], antituberculosis [41], and anticancer effects [19,43].

The toxicity of vanadium anticancer complexes presents another challenge and potential concern. Vanadium concentration in human blood plasma is reported in the range 0.2–15 nM, and this concentration changes upon administration of vanadium compounds [3]. However, according to human studies, the concentration of vanadium does not change linearly as the concentration of the treatment agent increases [44]. For example, several studies have shown that long-term administration of vanadium can cause accumulation in the bone. Still, other metal-based cancer treatments, such as protein/peptide vaccines for immunotherapy, use much more toxic metal adjuvants than vanadium, such as aluminum oxide salts [45,46].

In the last decade of vanadium anticancer research, many promising vanadium compounds for cancer treatment have been identified. These compounds include vanadium salts, oxovanadium coordination complexes, and polyoxidovanadates (POVs). In this review, we highlight recent advances in vanadium anticancer research over the last 5 years and identify key studies with other prevalent diseases.

2   ANTICANCER APPLICATIONS OF VANADIUM COMPOUNDS

Vanadium salts were first reported to have anticancer properties in 1965 [8,47], followed by a report in 1986 that vanadocene, an organovanadium compound that has a vanadium ion sandwiched between two cyclopentadienyl rings, has antitumoral effects [8,48]. Vanadocene is the first non-oxo organovanadium species to have reported anticancer effects [3]. Vanadocene has been shown to induce apoptosis in HepG2 (human liver) cells, yet its mechanism of action remains unknown.

Recent studies indicate that vanadocene does not cause primary DNA damage, meaning that its mechanism of action is different from the leading metal-based cancer treatment, cisplatin [49].

These initial reports have inspired further research into vanadium-based anticancer agents. In general, vanadium anticancer compounds induce apoptosis by disrupting cellular metabolism through generation of ROS, DNA damage, and alteration of organelles and signaling pathways [3,17,50,51]. The following sections will explore different classes of anticancer vanadium compounds, including vanadium salts, coordination complexes, and POVs, and modes of administration of these agents.

2.1 VANADIUM COORDINATION COMPLEXES

2.1.1 V(IV/V) Oxo Complexes

Vanadium oxo complexes contain one oxo group and constitute most of the novel vanadium anticancer agents reported over the last 5 years. Metvan ([$V^{IV}O(OSO_3)$ (phen)$_2$] where phen = 1,10-phenanthroline, Figure 2) is a well-known vanadium(IV) oxo complex that was initially reported for anticancer applications in the early 2000s [3]. Studies with metvan have recently suggested that it is a promising multitargeted anticancer complex with apoptosis-inducing activity in leukemia, glioblastoma, myeloma, and solid tumor cells [52]. However, metvan undergoes hydrolysis in both PBS and MEM media, which is confirmed by UV-Vis and EPR speciation data at pH 7.4, suggesting that the complex hydrolyzes upon entering cells. Therefore, recent studies have revisited its cytotoxicity [53]. The toxicity of both complex and ligand was investigated, and the study established that the toxicity of the complex is mainly caused by the phen ligand, not vanadium itself, thus bringing into question the potential application of metvan as a cancer therapeutic in future studies [53].

Vanadium oxo complexes with antioxidant flavonoid ligands (Figure 2) have been explored because of the potential that the resulting complexes would be very active [55,57–61]. Several flavonoid ligands form complexes that affect gene expression, metabolic pathways, and DNA damage [59]. Flavonoids also inhibit several ROS-producing enzymes, including monooxygenase, cyclooxygenase, lipoxygenase, NADH, and phospholipase [59]. Vanadium complexes reported

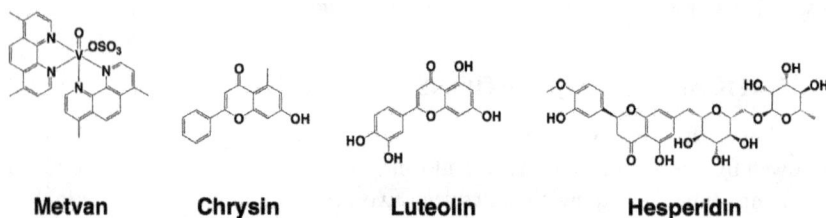

Metvan   Chrysin   Luteolin   Hesperidin

FIGURE 2   Oxovanadium complexes and flavonoid ligands reported for anticarcinogenic vanadium complexes [54–57].

with flavonoid ligands include quercetin, hesperidin, morin, silibinin, and chrysin [55,57–59,62]. These complexes are cytotoxic against several cancer cell lines. This cytotoxicity is attributed to the pro-oxidant nature of flavonoid ligands and the ability of the complexes to generate ROS [59]. The nature of the vanadium-flavonoid complexes has been characterized by several techniques, including FTIR, UV-Vis, and elemental analysis (Table 1); however, crystal structures of these complexes remain elusive. Interestingly, some of the vanadium-flavonoid complexes are less cytotoxic than the corresponding ligands, such as chrysin, suggesting that some structural differences exist that affect the anticancer potential of these materials. A better understanding of these differences would be desirable before further exploration of these systems for cancer treatment.

Several oxovanadium(IV) complexes have been reported as promising agents for photodynamic therapy (PDT) due to their near-IR d-d light absorption [6]. The complexes with N,N-donor dipyridophenazine (dppz) ligand were reported in 2007, showing a weak d–d band around 840 and 700 nm and another one around 470 nm [66]. The curcumin oxovanadium complexes have also been of interest for ROS production and DNA binding [67,68]. The oxovanadium curcumin complexes absorb light around 450 nm due to pi-pi* transitions and 720 nm due to their MC bands, resulting in a good Type I PDT effect with IC_{50} values of 10 µM under visible light irradiation in HeLa cells [67,68]. Oxovanadium(IV) complexes with BODIPY ligands are the most promising PDT agents upon irradiation at 535 nm due to the emission properties of BODIPY that allow for cellular imaging [69,70]. A recent study has also reported several oxovanadium(V) Schiff base complexes that accumulate in breast cancer cell lines and show cytotoxicity [71]. A novel imidazo[4,5-f] [1,10]- phenanthroline oxidovanadium(IV) complex had an IC_{50} of 8.2 µM in human keratinocytes (HaCaT) under visible light irradiation [72]. The representative oxovanadium(IV) complexes for PDT are shown in Figure 3. Overall, the development of V(IV) complexes for PDT is an emerging area where a careful design of the ligands may result in vanadium complexes with favorable properties for both PDT and cancer treatment. For example, novel two-dimensional (2D) vanadium-based nanosheets (Vanadene, V NSs) with polyvalent surfaces (V^{IV}/V^{V}) and high biodegradability were prepared by a liquid-phase exfoliation strategy [73]. The polyvalent surface entailed with multiple capabilities to modulate TME through GSH consumption and O_2 production via V^V and to catalyze a Fenton-like reaction to produce OH under mild conditions via V^{IV}. The V-NSs-based nanocatalyst can be slowly degraded into non-toxic species, enabling it to be innocuously eliminated from the body after completing tumor eradication by single drug injection and single NIR irradiation.

2.1.1.1 *Vanadium Schiff Base Complexes: V^{IV}, V^V, and Mono and Dioxo Complexes*

Schiff base ligands provide scaffolds that support diverse coordination modes and participate in many biological activities, making them desirable in catalysis, as fluorescence sensors, and in drug development [3]. Vanadium Schiff base complexes,

TABLE 1

Vanadium(IV/V) Flavonoid Complexes, Their Reported Characterization, and Observed Biological Activities of the Complexes

Complex	Ligand	Reported Characterization	Reported Anticancer Properties	Ref.
[VO(apigenin)(H$_2$O)$_2$] Cl	apigenin	Elemental analysis, TGA, diffuse reflection	Lung (A549) and cervix HeLa cancer cells	[61]
[VO(dios)(OH)$_3$] Na$_3$·6H$_2$O	diosmin	Elemental analysis, UV-Vis, TGA	Lung (A549) and breast (T47D, SKBR3 and MDAMB231) cancer cell lines	[63]
[VO(luteolin)$_2$]	luteolin	UV-Vis, FTIR, ESI-MS	N/A, ROS formation was tracked using 1-diphenyl-2-picrylhydrazyl (DPPH)	[56]

(Continued)

TABLE 1 (Continued)
Vanadium(IV/V) Flavonoid Complexes, Their Reported Characterization, and Observed Biological Activities of the Complexes

Complex	Ligand	Reported Characterization	Reported Anticancer Properties	Ref.
$[VO(Quer)_2EtOH]_n$	quercetin	UV-Vis, elemental analysis	Osteoblastic cell cultures: normal (MC3T3E1) and tumoral (UMR106),	[58]
$[VO(Hesp)(OH)_3]$ Na$_4$·3H$_2$O (VOHesp)	hesperidin	FTIR, elemental analysis	Rat osteosarcoma (UMR106) and human colon adeno-carcinoma (Caco-2)	[57]
$[VO(mor)_2H_2O]$·5H$_2$O (VOmor)	morin	UV-Vis, FTIR, elemental analysis, diffuse reflection	Osteoblast (UMR106 and MC3T3E1), breast tumor (T47D and SKBR3) and breast epithelial cell lines	[62]

(Continued)

TABLE 1 (*Continued*)
Vanadium(IV/V) Flavonoid Complexes, Their Reported Characterization, and Observed Biological Activities of the Complexes

Complex	Ligand	Reported Characterization	Reported Anticancer Properties	Ref.
[VO(rutin)₂]	Rutin	¹H NMR, ESI-MS, FTIR, UV-Vis	Oral subacute toxicity study in balb/c mice. Mortality observed at a dose of 120 mg/kg	[64]
[VO(chrysin)₂EtOH]₂		FTIR, elemental analysis	Human osteosarcoma cell line (MG-63)	[55,65]

chrysin

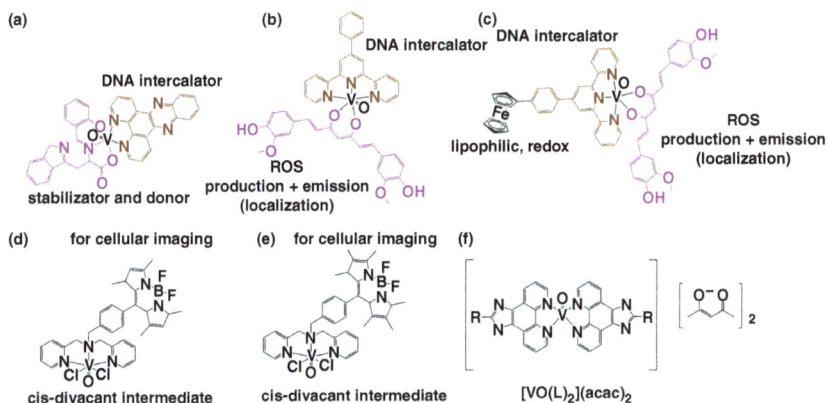

FIGURE 3 Representative oxovanadium(IV) complexes for PDT.

however, are susceptible to hydrolysis under physiological conditions. Thus, novel delivery methods for those complexes may be required for further development of these compounds for therapeutic purposes [74]. The class of vanadium Schiff base complexes continues to grow due to their convenient synthesis and characterization, in addition to the fact that the framework stabilizes complexes including metal ions in high oxidation states. Schiff base ligands have been used for decades to model the coordination mode and reactivity of vanadium in biological systems in studies exploring the chemistry of haloperoxidase enzymes [75].

In the last 5 years, oxovanadium(IV/V) Schiff base complexes for application as anticancer agents have been reported. While some of the reported complexes have $IC_{50} > 50$ µM or have comparable cytotoxicity to cisplatin (refer to [76–79]), several novel vanadium Schiff base complexes have high cytotoxicity, making them promising anticancer agents (Figure 4) [80]. For example, a newly synthesized oxovanadium complex $(HNEt_3)[V^VO_2L]$ where L = H_2L = 4-((E)-(2-hydroxy-5-nitrophenylimino)methyl)benzene-1,3-diol] has demonstrated moderate cytotoxicity against colon cancer cell lines (HT-29, $IC_{50} = 9.09 \pm 0.03$ µM) [81] and low cytotoxicity against mouse embryonic fibroblast (NIH-3T3, $IC_{50} = 79.77 \pm 4.00$ µM) cancer cell lines [81]. Vanadium(IV) naphthoylhydrazone complex (Figure 4a) has been found to be a promising multitargeted anticancer complex with high cytotoxicity in lung (H1299, $IC_{50} = 7.0$ µM), breast (MCF7, $IC_{50} = 0.73$ µM), and colon (HCT116, $IC_{50} = 1.12$ µM) cancer cell lines [82]. A new series of vanadium dinuclear complexes of tridentate halogen-substituted Schiff bases with the $O \rightarrow V^{IV} = O \rightarrow V^{IV} = O$ core (Figure 4b) has been evaluated in ovarian (A2780), breast (MCF7), and prostate (PC3) cancer cells at 48 hours [83]. The results with these multitargeted anticancer compounds have shown that these complexes are highly cytotoxic, with IC_{50} values in the range of 3.9–17.2 µM [83].

VO(hntdtsc)(NPIP) shown in Figure 4c significantly inhibited tumor growth and induced the apoptosis of cancer cells in mouse xenograft models, according to the results of *in vivo* image detection, H&E pathological examination,

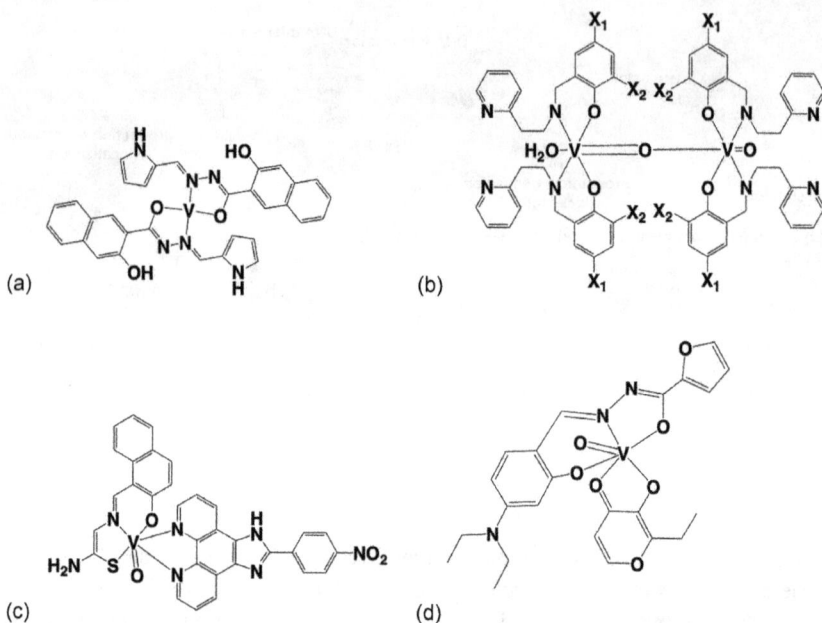

FIGURE 4 Oxidovanadium(IV/V) Schiff base complexes with reported anticancer properties.

and immunohistochemical detection of p16/Ki-67 protein expression [80]. This complex was tested in several cell lines and was found to have an IC_{50} of 1.09 μM in HeLa cells, 4.51 μM in BIU-87 cells, and 7.61 μM in SPC-A-1 cells. An oxidovanadium [$V^VOL(ema)$] complex was synthesized using tridentate ONO donor ligands (Figure 4d). The *in vitro* cytotoxicity activity was tested against lung (A549) and colon (HT-29) cancer cell lines and a non-cancerous mouse fibroblast (NIH-3T3) cell line. The anticancer activity was manifested in an IC_{50} value of 4.4 ± 0.1 μM against the HT-29 cell line [84]. The complex induces cell cycle arrest at the G2/M phase, and a dose-dependent cell apoptosis is triggered, as measured by the cell apoptosis analysis via flow cytometry and confocal microscopy assays. The complex targets the mitochondria by disrupting the mitochondrial membrane potential and causing overproduction of intracellular ROS, eventually leading to induced cell apoptosis [84]. Overall, recent reports have introduced several interesting oxovanadium(IV/V) complexes, although rigorous cytotoxicity assays are necessary to assure that the scaffolds used are not contributing to the observed cytotoxicity in cancer cell lines.

Vanadium(V) catecholate complexes are a subclass of vanadium Schiff base complexes with reported anticancer properties (Figure 5) [85–87]. The studies by the Crans and Lay groups have shown that bulky hydrophobic substituents on the catecholate ligand increase hydrolytic stability and cytotoxicity in T98g (glioblastoma multiforme) cells, as these complexes readily hydrolyze under physiological conditions [86,87]. The modest hydrolytic stability makes

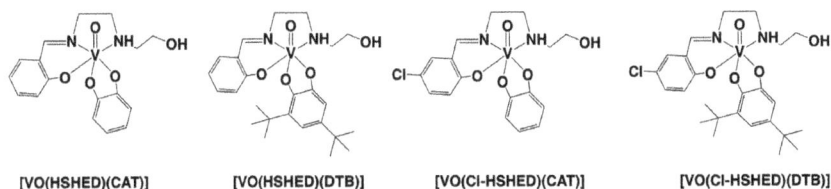

[VO(HSHED)(CAT)]   [VO(HSHED)(DTB)]   [VO(Cl-HSHED)(CAT)]   [VO(Cl-HSHED)(DTB)]

FIGURE 5 Structures of vanadium(V) catecholate complexes as potential agents for glioblastoma treatment where HSHED is N-(salicylideneaminato)-N'-(2-hydroxyethyl)-1, 2-ethanediamine, CAT – catechol and DTB – di-*tert*-butylcatechol [74,85–87].

vanadium(V) catecholate complexes suitable agents to treat glioblastoma via intratumoral injections (ITIs); they are sufficiently stable to be administered but are very reactive with tumors before any diffusion takes place [74,86]. The spectroscopic properties and cytotoxicities of several non-halogenated and halo-genated complexes abbreviated VO(HSHED), where HSHED stands for *N*-(salic ylideneaminato)-*N'*-(2-hydroxyethyl)-1,2-ethanediamine, have been reported in addition to their anticancer properties in T98g (glioblastoma multiforme), A549 (lung), PANC-1 (pancreatic), and SW1353 (bone chondrosarcoma) cell lines. The [VO(HSHED)(DTB)] and [VO(Cl-HSHED) (DTB)] complexes, where DTB stands for di-*tert*-butylcatechol (IC$_{50}$ = 2.5 ± 0.1 and 4.1 ± 0.5 µM, respectively), have been found to be most cytotoxic toward cancer cells but less toxic toward normal cells and most hydrolytically stable due to the steric bulk of the *tert*-butyl substituents on the catecholate ligand [85–87].

Dioxovanadium Schiff base complexes, a much smaller subclass of vana-dium Schiff base complexes, have two oxo groups and have also been reported. A *cis*-dioxovanadium species with the formula (HNEt$_3$)[V^{V}O$_2$L] was reported to be highly cytotoxic in colon cancer cell lines (HT-29 cells, IC$_{50}$ = 8.56 ± 0.62 µM) while being non-toxic to normal cell lines (NIH-3T3 cells, IC$_{50}$ = 67.8 ± 5.48 µM), making it a promising treatment for colon cancer [81]. Another dioxovanadium species, with a dimeric structure and the formula [(V^{V}O$_2$)$_2$(pedf)$_2$], is a promis-ing multitargeted anticancer treatment with relatively low cytotoxicity in lung cancer (A549 cells, IC$_{50}$ = 64.2 µM) and in human skin carcinoma (A431 cells, IC$_{50}$ = 56.3 µM) cell lines [88].

Overall, this section summarizes the diversity of structures and applications of vanadium(IV/V) Schiff base complexes for different types of cancer. Rigorous assay studies are much needed to evaluate whether the toxicity of newly synthesized vanadium(IV/V) Schiff base complexes is attributed to the complex or the free ligand.

2.1.2 V^V Dioxo Complexes

Vanadium(V) dipicolinates contain the *cis*-dioxo moiety and have the general formula [VO$_2$dipic-X]$^-$. Vanadium(V) dipicolinates are well-known coordination complexes with antidiabetic properties [13,15,89] and are also reported to exert anticancer properties by enhancing the effects of oncolytic viruses (Figure 6) [13,89,90]. Oncolytic viruses are Food and Drug Administration –approved for the

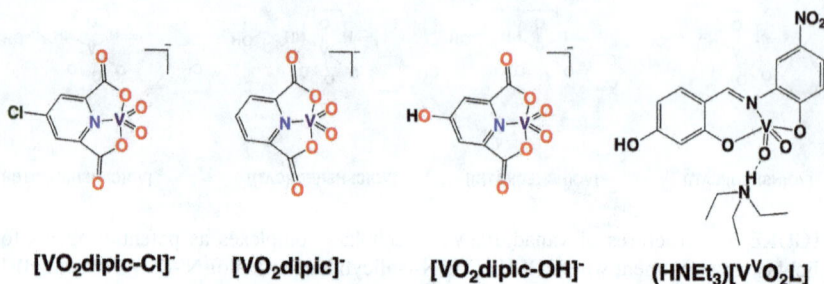

FIGURE 6   Representative dioxovanadium anticancer complexes [13,81,90].

treatment of advanced melanoma in both the U.S. and Europe [91]. Vanadium salts and complexes have been chosen due to their reported immunostimulatory and anticancer effects. Three vanadium(V) dipicolinate derivatives, [VO$_2$dipic-X]$^-$, where X = H, Cl, and OH, were tested in combination with oncolytic viruses, non-pathogenic DNA rhabidoviruses that preferentially infect and kill cancer cells by inducing antitumor immunity [90]. Vanadium(V) dipicolinates enhance the viral spread in 786-0 cells at the same magnitude of viral enhancement, as is reported for vanadium salts and vanadium(V) dipicolinates. Similarly, vanadium citrate complexes were investigated and also found to enhance oncolytic viruses [92]. The immunomodulatory mechanism of vanadate has been recently reported by Wong and coworkers [93], which indicates that vanadate regulates STAT1 and STAT2 heterodimers through the epidermal growth factor receptor (EGFR) to modulate the interferon (IFN) response, which consequentially results in the replication of oncolytic viruses [93]. The reports of vanadium coordination complexes enhancing the effects of oncolytic viruses open the possibilities of a promising efficient anticancer treatment.

2.1.3   Non-Oxovanadium Complexes

As described earlier, non-oxovanadium complexes include vanadocenes, a class of organometallic compounds that have a vanadium ion sandwiched between two cyclopentadienyl rings [48]. Vanadocene is the first non-oxo organovanadium species to have reported anticancer effects [3]. Vanadocene has been shown to induce apoptosis in HepG2 (human liver) cells, yet its mechanism of action remains unknown. Recent studies indicate that vanadocene does not cause primary DNA damage, meaning that its mechanism of action is different from cisplatin [49].

A recent study has reported non-oxovanadium tridentate ONO Schiff base complexes with promising inhibitory activities (IC$_{50}$ = 19.0 μM) of lysine-specific demethylase 1, an enzyme associated with the progress and oncogenesis of multiple human cancers (Figure 7) [94]. A series of structurally similar complexes has been reported shortly thereafter, with the lead complex of the series being highly cytotoxic in gastric (MCG803, IC$_{50}$ = 2.69 ± 0.56 μM), breast (MCF7, IC$_{50}$ = 4.52 ± 0.65 μM), and liver (HepG2, IC$_{50}$ = 5.50 ± 0.74 μM) cancer cell lines and drug-resistant esophageal squamous cell carcinoma (EC109, IC$_{50}$ = 7.21 ± 0.85 μM) [95].

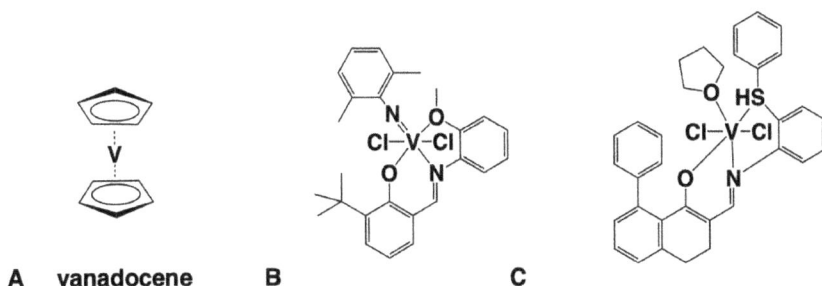

A   vanadocene   B   C

FIGURE 7   Representative vanadium anticancer complexes.

2.2   VANADIUM SALTS

Vanadium salts are well-known and well-studied antidiabetic agents, some of which have been studied in phase I and II clinical trials ($VOSO_4$ and $NaVO_3$) [7,96]. Consequently, the research focus has recently shifted toward anticancer applications of vanadium salts (Figure 8) [91,97,98].

Vanadium(IV/V) salts, such as vanadyl sulfate ($VOSO_4$), sodium orthovanadate (Na_3VO_4), and sodium metavanadate ($NaVO_3$), are being used in several anticancer studies (Figure 8). $VOSO_4$ is often a positive control that is used frequently. Recently, $VOSO_4$ and $NaVO_3$ have been tested in combination with oncolytic viruses [92]. The first study documented that all salts robustly enhance the spread of oncolytic viruses, which led to subsequent studies with vanadium coordination complexes [90,99]. The combination of vanadyl sulfate and Newcastle disease virus has been administered via ITIs and has proven effective in melanoma and murine prostate cancer models [91]. $NaVO_3$ has been reported to exhibit antiproliferative effects in the human pancreatic cancer cell line AsPC-1 by inducing the activation of both PI3K/AKT and MAPK/ERK signaling pathways dose- and time-dependently [98]. Sodium metavanadate has also been tested in a murine breast cancer model, both *in vitro* and *in vivo*. The data have shown that $NaVO_3$ inhibits proliferation of murine breast cancer cells 4T1 with IC_{50} values of 8.19

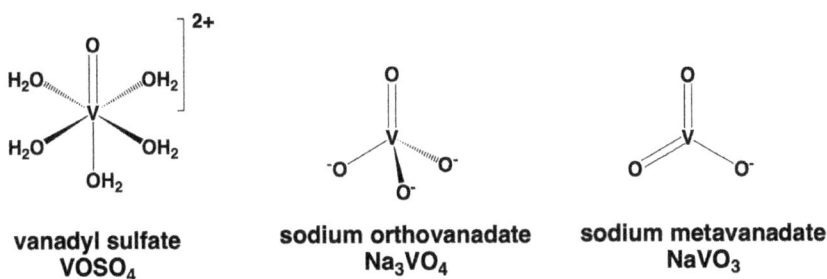

vanadyl sulfate
$VOSO_4$

sodium orthovanadate
Na_3VO_4

sodium metavanadate
$NaVO_3$

FIGURE 8   Structures of vanadium(IV/V) salts studied for their anticancer applications. These structures represent the anionic forms of the respective oxovanadates.

and 1.92 μM at 24 and 48 hours, respectively [97]. The study has also reported the underlying mechanism of the inhibition activity, where NaVO$_3$ increases the ROS levels in a concentration-dependent way, arrests cells at the G2/M phase, diminishes the mitochondrial membrane potential, and promotes the progress of apoptosis [97]. NaVO$_3$ has also exhibited dose-dependent anticancer activity in breast cancer-bearing mice that led to the shrinkage of tumor volume by about 50% [97]. Overall, the studies with vanadium salts have established a foundation for the development of more efficient vanadium-based anticancer therapeutics.

2.3 POLYOXIDOVANADATES

POVs are polyanionic vanadium-oxygen clusters and a subclass of polyoxido-metalates (POMs), which is a class of compounds consisting of group V and VI metal-oxide clusters [19]. The first report of the anticancer activity of a POM was published in 1965, and the field has grown significantly since then [19]. The number of papers regarding the use of POMs for anticancer applications has increased sevenfold over the last decade, with about 10% of publications covering anticancer applications of POVs. POVs have been reported to demonstrate biological activities against diabetes, cancer, bacteria, and viral diseases [19,41,100]. Two decavanadate derivatives, (H$_2$tmen)$_3$[V$_{10}$O$_{28}$] (tmen = N,N,N^0,N^0-tetramethylethylenediamine) and (H$_2$en)$_3$[V$_{10}$O$_{28}$] (en = ethylenediamine), have been found highly effective against human lung carcinoma (A549; IC$_{50}$ = 4.3 ± 0.3 and 1.5 ± 0.1 μM, respectively) [101]. The clusters, however, have been found to be highly cytotoxic to normal hepatocytes (IC$_{50}$ = 6.5 ± 0.6 and 7.2 ± 0.7 μM, respectively) [101]. For more information regarding the anticancer applications of POMs and POV, refer to the recent reviews [19,43].

2.4 NOVEL MODES OF ADMINISTRATION OF VANADIUM ANTICANCER COMPOUNDS

The mode of administration is highly dependent on the compound and its potential application. Due to its non-invasive nature, cost effectiveness, and patient convenience and compliance, oral administration has traditionally been the most preferred method to administer vanadium compounds [102]. The compounds are often added to food in animal studies or in some carriers that generally improve the absorption of the drug significantly. Oral administration of vanadium complexes and salts, such as BMOV, VOSO$_4$, and NaVO$_3$, has been most extensively investigated in phase I and II clinical trials for diabetes treatment [7,14]. The oral administration of organovanadium species such as BMOV and BEOV is advantageous as the bioavailability of vanadium increases threefold compared to the vanadium salts [7,14]. However, the distribution and cell uptake are much lower than desired, causing a higher systemic concentration needed for treatment. BEOV, an organovanadium(IV) antidiabetic drug studied in phase I and II clinical trials, went off patent in 2011, which unfortunately put the studies exploring the safety of oral administration of vanadium compounds on hold [14].

Different methods of administration of vanadium compounds are used for the treatment of cancer. Since cancer can be terminal, more aggressive methods of administration are generally developed and used in the clinic. The following section describes modes of administration of vanadium anticancer compounds, such as nanoparticles and ITIs. These methods provide targeted delivery and show a significant reduction of cancerous tumors. The resulting reduced systemic toxicity to normal tissues is particularly desirable.

2.4.1   Oral Administration via Lipid Nanoparticles (LNPs)

Lipid nanoparticles are used both as a diagnostic tool and as a drug carrier for specific organs and tissues. Among different types of nanotransporters, lipid nanotransporters are most frequently used in medicine due to their high biocompatibility, controlled release, and ability to encapsulate both hydrophilic and hydrophobic species [103]. Lipid nanotransporters are increasingly used for the delivery of highly cytotoxic platinum metallodrugs to reduce overall systemic toxicity [103,104]. Several delivery methods have been reported for vanadium anticancer agents, including micelles, liposomes, inorganic nanoparticles, polymeric nanoparticles, and proteins (albumin, ferritin) [74,105]. A recent study has reported using four different LNP formulations to encapsulate metvan, one of the most well-known vanadium(IV) anticancer complexes [54]. An optimization process concluded that the desirable formulation consisted of 505.0 mg of myristyl myristate and 4.0% p/v of Pluronic F128 surfactant in an aqueous medium. The biological studies have shown that the LNP formulation decreases the cell viability of osteosarcoma (MG-63 cells) in the MTT assay from 90% (metvan at 25 μM loading) to 30% (metvan-LNP formulation at 25 μM metvan loading) [54]. There is no doubt that such approaches will significantly enhance the efficacy of the potential anticancer agents and allow for a reduction in the systemic concentration needed for treatment.

2.4.2   Intratumoral Injections

ITIs provide a method of procedure that is increasingly applied in the clinic due to their novel mode of delivery of highly cytotoxic metal-based anticancer complexes (Figure 9) [74]. The ongoing and recent clinical trials with ITIs use established Pt-based anticancer drugs, such as cisplatin, carboplatin, and oxaliplatin [74]. Two related techniques, convection-enhanced delivery [106–108] and pressurized intraperitoneal aerosolized chemotherapy [109,110], are being developed to increase the cytotoxic drug concentration within the tumor and to decrease the concentration outside the tumor and in the blood. The concept of using ITIs has been recently proposed for relatively unstable, non-innocent oxidovanadium(V) catecholate complexes. The complexes consist of a tridentate Schiff base and a redox-active catecholate ligand (Figure 9). Previous studies have shown that the catecholate complexes with bulky hydrophobic substituents on the

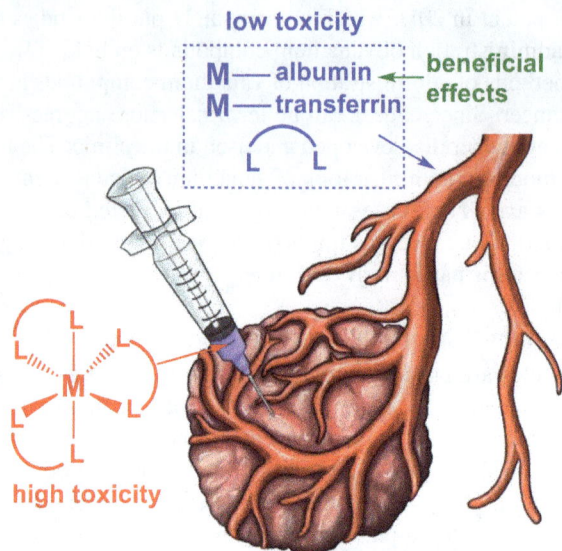

FIGURE 9 The principle of the use of reactive and unstable metal complexes in intra-tumoral injections. Designations: M is the metal ion; and L are the ligands. (The image was reproduced from Ref. [74] under the Creative Commons Attribution-Share Alike 4.0 Unported license (https://creativecommons.org/licenses/by- sa/4.0/deed.en)).

catecholate ligand are the most suitable agents for ITIs due to their high cyto-toxicity and relatively short lifetimes in media (half-life = 30 seconds at 37°C). The hydrophobic bulk of the catecholate ligand increases hydrolytic stability in media and uptake into cancer cell monolayers. Consequently, this causes high cytotoxicity in cancer cell monolayers, which has been reported for the lead com-plex of the catecholate series, [VO(HSHED)(DTB)] (IC_{50} 1–4 µM in 72-hour treatments). Additionally, previous studies have shown that decomposition side products of the catecholate complexes, such as V-Tf adducts, are non-toxic and, in some cases, can have neuroprotective and neurostimulatory effects [74].

ITIs have also been proposed for other vanadium(V) complexes and vana-dium salts. One of the recent studies has reported using ITIs of $VOSO_4$ and Newcastle disease virus [91]. This combination therapy was effective in mela-noma and murine prostate cancer models [91]. Another study has reported using ITIs of a novel vanadium(V) nanocomplex for PDT [111]. The complex consists of vanadyl ions chelated with tannic acid and silk sericin, a biocompatible protein. The vanadyl(V) nanocomplex has been injected into tumors 7 and 10 days after tumor inoculation, followed by PDT treatment. The results have demonstrated the enhancement of photothermal-induced cancer immunotherapy to inhibit primary tumor metastasis and recurrence by the novel vanadyl(V) nanocomplex [111].

In summary, ITIs and related methods are a new and promising avenue of vanadium anticancer research that are currently used as palliative methods for late-stage cancers. The evidence from the ongoing clinical trials shows that these administration methods will soon be employed in modern medicine. Importantly, these methods allow the administration of hydrolytically unstable and cytotoxic hydrophobic complexes, as well as vanadium salts. When optimized, the ITIs maximize the concentration of cytotoxic species in the target tumor and reduce the concentrations outside the tumor and in the blood. Overall, this results in a decrease in the systemic concentration of the drug and significantly lower toxicity.

3   APPLICATIONS OF VANADIUM FOR THE TREATMENT OF DIABETES AND CARDIOVASCULAR PROBLEMS

Diabetes mellitus is a complex disease classified into Types 1 and 2 with distinct clinical features. Type 1 is an autoimmune disease where beta cells in the pancreas cannot produce insulin, while in Type 2 diabetes, the body is either partially or completely resistant to insulin, unable to produce sufficient amounts of insulin, or a combination of both [112]. Both types of diabetes mellitus cause chronic hyperglycemia, which, when uncontrolled, has dramatic consequences for multiple essential organs, such as the cardiovascular system and its function [112,113]. Vanadium salts and coordination compounds have a long history of normalizing elevated blood glucose levels [7,13,16]. Indeed, several compounds have undergone phase I and II clinical trials, although most of these studies were done at a time when the requirements for such studies were more lenient and did not require as many subjects or time of the clinical trial [3,7,14]. However, as described below, some of the same enzymes and metabolic pathways are impacted in cancer and diabetes, so some of the studies carried out on both diseases are relevant to each other [18,96].

3.1   REPORTS OF ANTIDIABETIC VANADIUM COMPLEXES

Recent studies demonstrating the antidiabetic effects of vanadium compounds report a decrease in elevated blood glucose levels *in vivo* and *in vitro*, meaning that the recent studies [114–120] confirm the studies reported previously [7,14,15,18,19,21,96]. The following section describes *in vitro* studies, and animal studies are described in Section 5.

Type 2 diabetic patients with hyperglycemia showed increased oxidative stress and free radical-mediated lipid peroxidation [121–123], which may facilitate the development of micro- and macrovascular complications [124–126]. Compounds that modulate lipid peroxidation and oxidative stress and have antioxidant potential may, in part, contribute to improving the metabolic health of patients with diabetes [127]. For example, oxidative stress in the liver and muscle tissues of alloxan-induced diabetic rats was treated with $(H_2Metf)_3[V_{10}O_{28}]$ (metformin-decavanadate, MV_{10}), resulting in decreased levels of SOD and CAT activity [114–116,128]. Furthermore, lipid peroxidation markers and other effects were normalized similarly to treatment with insulin, whereas metformin alone showed fewer effects.

Vanadium compounds were reported to activate Akt signaling and tyrosine phosphorylation through inhibition of PTPs in CHO cells containing the human insulin receptor (CHO-HIR cells) [129]. Furthermore, organovanadium complexes and vanadium salts have also been reported to stimulate glucose transport in an insulin-deficient cardiac system. These reports confirm similar earlier reports with other vanadium compounds [21,130].

The PTP associated with the antidiabetic effects of vanadium compounds is protein phosphatase 1B (PTP1B). It was found that upon cell mutation and phosphatase removal, the cells are no longer affected by vanadium compounds [21,130,131]. Recent studies were done with this phosphatase, including measuring the inhibition constant of some acac-derived vanadium complexes [118] to complement the work reviewed preciously [21,130,131]. Prior to this work, it was expected that a similar transition state for the hydrolysis of alkyl phosphates and peptide phosphates would be found for all phosphatases. The hydrolysis of a phosphate ester that is found after the S_N2 attack results in trigonal bipyramidal transition state complexes. Vanadate forms stable five-coordinate trigonal bipyramidal complexes and, accordingly, inhibits most phosphatases potently. Hence, the similarities of the active site for all phosphatases have led to the expectation that it was impossible to develop an inhibitor that was specific for any phosphatase. This expectation has become a dogma. However, recently, Yang and Crans developed a vanadate ester consisting of vanadate and an unnatural peptide ligand that was complementary to a cleft on PTP1B adjacent to the phosphate ester hydrolysis active site [132]. This vanadate ester is found to be an effective inhibitor for PTP1B. The approach for the development of this potent inhibitor is shown in Figure 10 [132]. Cell culture studies and animal studies in rats demonstrated that this inhibitor was not only specific in studies *in vitro* but, with the assistance of graphene quantum dots, was stabilized and able to enter cells through a lipid raft mechanism. Administration of such a system was found to be more effective than the bismaltolatoperoxovanadium(IV) complex that had been investigated in phase I and II clinical trials for the treatment of STZ-induced diabetic rats. These studies therefore show not only that the vanadium complex is a potent and selective inhibitor for PTP1B, but that in combination with graphene quantum dots, this vanadate ester can enter cells and normalize the diabetic animal.

Considering that the peptide analog bound to the vanadate can be readily changed, Yang and Crans replaced the initial peptide analog with a peptide that was specific for binding to the T-cell–specific phosphatase. This system was indeed found to no longer bind to PTP1B but instead to be specific for the T-cell PTP. This approach thus presented a new and general method for designing specific phosphatase inhibitors.

Vanadium complexes are also known to initiate signal transduction [35,37] and, accordingly, initiate a response in mammalian cells. Additionally, vanadium complexes are reported to mediate insulin activity and prompt the body to stabilize its insulin sensitivity. Some of these effects are due to the inhibition of PTPs. The inhibition of the PTPase that stimulates the insulin receptor tyrosine kinase activity will result in some cellular uptake of glucose [133]. In another study, Iglesias-González and coworkers found that BMOV was able to mimic the function of insulin in hyperglycemic rats [113]. This study, as well as many others

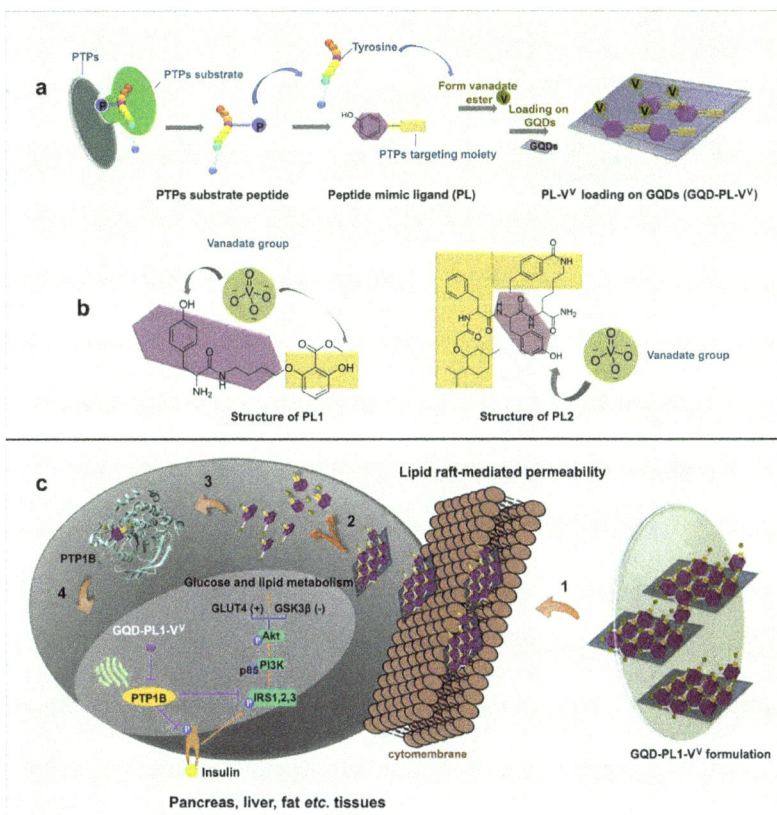

FIGURE 10 Concept and action of PTPs selective graphite quantum dot (GQD)-(peptide mimic ligand)-vanadate complex (GQD-PL1-VV). (a) Schematic diagram of GQD-(peptide mimic ligand)-vanadate complex; (b) Structure of the two inhibitors designed, one for PP1B (GQD-PL1-VV) and one for T-cell PTPase (GQD-PL2-VV); (c) Schematic diagram of cellular uptake and PTP1B inhibition of GQD-PL1-VV that were absorbed through lipid raft-mediated permeation (step 1). Then PL1-VV was released into the cytoplasm (step 2) and selectively bound to PTP1B (step 3) causing inhibition of PTP1B which trigger insulin signal transduction and downstream effects (step 4) (The figure is adapted with permission from Ref. [132], Copyright 2021, Wiley-VCH GmbH).

prior to it, shows that vanadium compounds can result in the same response as insulin [7,14,18,96,131,134].

3.2 Vanadium Compounds and Their Effects on the Cardiovascular System

In recent years, vanadium compounds have demonstrated efficacy in the treatment of a broad range of cardiovascular diseases, including myocardial ischemia, hypertension, and myocardial hypertrophy [113,129]. More specifically, vanadium compounds have shown potential for the treatment of metabolic syndrome and for the treatment of heart attacks. The following section describes vanadium compounds as prospective treatments for these cardiovascular diseases.

The impact of vanadium salts (Na_3VO_4 and $VOSO_4$) and complexes (bis(maltolato)oxovanadium and VO(OPT)) [135] on treating the effects of metabolic syndrome contributes to the improved cardiovascular function from vanadium treatment by multiple factors, including the increase of GLUT translocation to plasma membrane and glucose transport, activation of the PI3K/Akt pathway in cardiomyocytes, and endothelial NO synthase. The function is further improved by the decrease of hepatic triglyceride glucose intolerance, and pre-adipocyte differentiation through PPAR-γ and C/EBPs expression. The primary result of these effects is improved smooth muscle contractility and lowered blood pressure [133]. The impact of vanadium complexes on metabolic syndrome is also linked to the effect of vanadium on vascular muscles and blood vessels.

3.3   THE EFFECTS OF VANADIUM ON MYOCARDIAL INFARCTION (HEART ATTACKS)

The ability of vanadium compounds to inhibit PTPases has the potential to be cardioprotective and to also treat metabolic syndrome. The inhibition of a PTP by vanadate may result in the upregulation of protein kinase B (Akt), which is important in cardiac growth. Upregulating protein kinase B can prevent a heart attack and support recovery during the post-heart-attack period. Specifically, a pyridine-thiolato complex and a picolinato-bis(peroxide)vanadium(V) complex have been reported to have significant cardioprotective effects in animal studies [136].

Furthermore, vanadium complexes have recently been used to determine their efficacy in cardioprotection, especially for the prevention of myocardial infarction (heart attacks). Vanadium complexes present potential as key inhibitors of lipid phosphatase and tensin homolog on chromosome ten (PTEN). The inhibition of this enzyme plays a significant role in limiting heart attack size and improving heart function after a heart attack episode [137]. For example, Keyes and coworkers examined how bisperoxovanadium [BpV(HOpic)] can inhibit PTEN genes to improve ventricular function after a heart attack [137]. Bisperoxovanadium [BpV(HOpic)] was found to reduce the size of the heart attack and the accompanying side effects. The study found that BpV protects cardiomyocytes against simulated ischemia and ischemia-reperfusion injury, presumably through inhibition of PTEN [137].

4   REACTIVE OXYGEN SPECIES, LIPID PEROXIATION IN DISEASE, AND OXIDATIVE STRESS

Vanadium is known to impact the formation of ROS, lipid peroxidation, and oxidative stress [17]. Depending on conditions and the nature of the vanadium species, vanadium compounds have been found to induce [17,138–140] or decrease [17,141–143] ROS. The effects are observed when using lipid peroxidation markers such as malondialdehyde, thiobarbituric acid, or 4-hydroxy-2-nonenal (4-HNE) [144–146]. However, the mode of action is complex, and vanadium can directly or indirectly have effects on ROS via Fenton reactions [147] or Haber-Weiss mechanisms [140,147]. For example, $VOSO_4$ is known to increase ROS formation faster than the effects of vanadate, consistent with the conversion of vanadate to vanadyl before the initiation of ROS. Furthermore, vanadate monomer and decavanadate are known to impact ROS differently [138,139]. Little has been done with exploring the effects of the speciation of vanadium complexes on ROS levels [17]. The difference in responses to simple salts and oxidovanadates suggests that the differences will be observed with vanadium complexes, particularly if speciation of the complexes is considered.

Oxidative stress, ROS, and lipid peroxidation have been implicated in diseases such as cancer, diabetes, and neurogenerative diseases [17]. Recent reports document similar effects caused by vanadium compounds both in cellular studies and in animal model systems, and future studies might reveal that those similar effects are not accidental. For example, coadministration of $VOSO_4$ with selenium tetrachloride ($SeCl_4$) significantly reduces the oxidative stress and lipid peroxidation levels obtained in studies with only the administration of $VOSO_4$ [148]. A better understanding of the impact of vanadium on lipid peroxidation and ROS formation will consequently help design better anticancer and antidiabetic treatments.

5 ANIMAL STUDIES WITH VANADIUM ANTICANCER AND ANTIDIABETIC COMPLEXES

The efficacy of several vanadium coordination complexes and salts was tested in human studies some time ago, mainly for the treatment of diabetes [149]. More recent analyses require longer studies and more subjects in the studies [3,149]. Several human studies have been recently reported to test the efficacy of vanadium. One large human study, involving approximately 1,500 human patients, demonstrated that low levels of vanadium in their diet are protective against the development of a metabolic disease, such as diabetes [150]. In a different study, higher vanadium content was observed in rejected kidneys and in cancerous kidneys [151]. In another study, vanadium coordination chemistry explained the pharmacokinetics and clinical response of administered vanadyl sulfate in Type 2 diabetic patients [44]. The study with 7,359 pregnant women enrolled at Wuhan Medical and Health Center, however, demonstrated that exposure to vanadium causes the highest risk of preterm births (defined as 37 weeks of completed gestation or less according to the World Health Organization) [152]. Of the 18 transition metal ions measured in the urine, vanadium, chromium, and zinc cause the highest risk of preterm births [152].

Numerous animal studies with vanadium compounds have been carried out over the years. The studies demonstrated the blood glucose-lowering effects of vanadium compounds [7,14,15,18,19,21,96]. Several complexes with blood glucose-lowering effects have been reported recently, including both known compounds [114–116] and novel complexes [117–120]. These studies showed that known complexes can be improved by modifications and applications of structure-activity relationships as novel vanadium complexes are continuously developed. Specifically, studies with the combination of decavanadate and metformin continue to show that the effect of the combination of these compounds is better than each compound separately in animal models other than the STZ-induced diabetic rats [114–116]. The new complexes included oxovanadium(IV) acac derivatives. One study of these derivatives showed that methyl imidazole complexes were *in vitro* inhibitors for PTP1B, and one of them was shown to normalize elevated blood glucose levels. A second study showed an oxovanadium(IV) acac derivative with a 3,4-diaminobenzoic acid complex had insulin-enhancing properties, although at a lower level than $VOSO_4$. Two studies with oxovanadium(IV) complexes administered oral gavage animal studies with a nitrogen-oxidovanadium(IV) and a sulfur-oxidovanadium(IV) complex, both showing improved effects compared to $VOSO_4$ and insulin. The results with these compounds are particularly noteworthy because both complexes have limited stability in aqueous solutions. Since the effects of the complexes were investigated using oral gavage administration, the complexes were intact when administered and for about 30 minutes after the administration.

Recently, two systematic reviews of vanadium were reported [132,149]. One of the reviews dealt with the analysis of publications on vanadium and diabetic dyslipidemia. Lipid levels are very sensitive to the diabetic condition. The electronic search identified 1,667 publications, of which 252 studies were considered further. The studies that did not meet inclusion criteria, including human studies and review articles, were excluded from the search. The search resulted in 124 articles for the analysis, 48 of which covered the studies carried out from 1989 to 2021. The studies were analyzed based on the vanadium compounds studied, separating out treatments with $VOSO_4$, vanadate (which include orthovanadate, metavanadate, and peroxovanadate), and coordination complexes. The systematic review of the 48 studies concluded that different forms of vanadium compounds do normalize the diabetes-induced alterations in lipid profile [149]. Considering that minor risk bias was found for most analyzed studies, it was confirmed that administration of both vanadium salts and coordination complexes could be beneficial in ameliorating lipid profile in diabetic animals and preventing vascular complications due to diabetes.

The second systematic review aimed to assess the effects of vanadium supplementation on inflammation and oxidative stress biomarkers in diabetes-induced animals, covering the period from 1990 to 2021. A total of 341 articles were evaluated, 42 of which were selected for inclusion. The vanadium compounds studied include $VOSO_4$, vanadate (which includes orthovanadate, metavanadate, and peroxovanadate), and several coordination complexes. The enzymatic activity of inflammatory biomarkers measured includes TNF-α, Il-6, hs-CRP, and caspase 3, as well as oxidative stress biomarkers including GSH, SOD,

GPx, GST, and GR. A minor risk of bias was reported based on SYRCLE's tool. Most of the studies confirmed the desirable properties of vanadium treatment on inflammatory and oxidative stress biomarkers in animals with Type 2 diabetes mellitus.

Much less has been done to explore vanadium treatments for animals with various types of cancer. Most of the reports involve tissue culture studies of primary cultures rather than animal experiments. Not only were different assays performed *in vitro* or *in vivo*, but different results were also obtained [37,38]. Vanadium compounds can activate different cancer signaling pathways and exert their antitumoral action. The MAPK/Erk, PI3K/Akt, caspase family, and JAK/Stat signaling pathways were stimulated by the vanadium compounds, prompting a cell cycle arrest, ROS production, and apoptosis toward different types of cancer cells. Nrf-2 was also activated by vanadium; however, in this case, it seemed to enhance the defense system and function as chemoprotective. The MAPK/Erk, PI3K/Akt, and caspase family and JAK/Stat signal and apoptosis toward different types of cancer cells [35,38].

The investigation of therapeutic applications of vanadium compounds must consider the toxicity of corresponding compounds, and some publications were recently reported [153–155]. One vanadium(V) catecholate complex, [VO(HSHED)(DTB)], which is currently investigated for cancer intratumoral treatment [86,87] was investigated in a recent animal study where the complex was administered at 300 mg/kg for 14 days [119]. The complex exhibited low oral acute toxicity and less than vanadate [119].

6   CONCLUSIONS AND OUTLOOK

Vanadium salts and complexes have been extensively considered as potential therapeutic agents for the past three decades. Initially, vanadium was considered as an antidiabetic agent; however, more recent studies focused on other effects of vanadium, particularly its anticancer effects. Vanadium(IV/V) coordination complexes, vanadium salts, and POVs gained attention for their antidiabetic applications, normalizing elevated blood glucose and lipid levels in diabetic mammals and humans. The ability of vanadium compounds to inhibit PTPs has been attributed to PTP1B; mutations of this PTPase eliminate the response of vanadium compounds. However, other mechanisms have been extensively investigated, including the interaction with blood proteins (transferrin, serum albumin, and immunoglobins), the redox state of the cells, and other metabolic pathways. Some of these metabolic pathways are also important for understanding the anticancer effects of vanadium. Thus, the studies that explored the antidiabetic pathways are now important for studies with vanadium anticancer agents.

Vanadium(IV/V) coordination complexes, vanadium salts, and POVs have gained increasing attention for anticancer applications in the past decade. Several metabolic and signaling pathways have been identified as targets and implicated in the mode of action of the vanadium compounds. Signaling pathways specific to vanadium compounds include those involving protein tyrosine kinases and

G-protein–coupled receptors, of which the effects of vanadium on the LHR have been studied most extensively. Vanadium also induces ROS formation, lipid peroxidation, and signal transduction. Vanadium compounds can also activate different cancer signaling pathways and exert their antitumoral action. The MAPK/Erk, PI3K/Akt, and caspase family and JAK/Stat signaling pathways were stimulated by the vanadium compounds, prompting a cell cycle arrest, ROS production, and apoptosis toward different types of cancer cells. Nrf-2 was also activated by vanadium; however, in this case, it seemed to enhance the defense system and function as chemoprotective. The MAPK/Erk, PI3K/Akt, and caspase family and JAK/Stat signal and apoptosis toward different types of cancer cells [35,38]. Some signaling pathways are inactivated by vanadium compounds and include the FAK, TGF-B/EMT, Notch-1, and autophagy signaling pathways. This inhibition could potentially result in cell arrest and apoptosis, a decrease in cellular migration and adhesions, FAK signaling pathway, autophagy signaling pathway, TGFbeta-EMT signaling pathway, and Notch-1-signaling pathway. These processes are important for cellular processes and are believed to exhibit tumor suppressor effects.

Vanadium anticancer complexes are structurally diverse and can be used to treat different types of cancer. Oxovanadium(IV/V) and dioxovanadium(IV/V) Schiff base complexes, in particular, have been the most growing classes of vanadium anticancer complexes for the past 5 years. These complexes support structural diversity and the ability to stabilize vanadium in physiologically relevant oxidation states IV and V. Oxovanadium(IV) complexes have also been investigated for PDT applications due to their photocytotoxicity in several cancer cell lines. The coordination complexes oxovanadium(V) dipicolinate and chlorodipicolinate complexes have been reported as oncolytic virotherapeutic agents, that combat cancer cell growth. VOSO4 is similarly a potent agent in this regard.

The development of modes of delivery of cytotoxic anticancer compounds, including vanadium(IV/V) complexes and salts, is important, and here we describe such applications of LNP carriers and ITIs which allow the delivery of the complexes to cancerous tissues with minimal damage to normal cells. Vanadium complexes continue to be explored for their antidiabetic applications and prevention of cardiovascular complications. Future development of vanadium-based therapeutics should also include considerations about their administration and stability, overall toxicity, and modes of action in the early stages of development.

ACKNOWLEDGMENTS

DCC thanks Colorado State University and the Arthur Cope Foundation, managed by the American Chemical Society, for funds.

ABBREVIATIONS AND DEFINITIONS

acac   acetylacetonate
BMOV   bis(maltolato)oxovanadium(IV)
ITIs   intratumoral injections

LHR	luteinizing hormone receptor
Metf	metformin
PDT	photodynamic therapy
PTP	protein tyrosine phosphatase
ROS	reactive oxygen species
SARS	severe acute respiratory syndrome coronavirus
STZ	streptozotocin
V_1	vanadate monomer ($VO_4{}^{3-}$)
V_{10}	decavanadate ($[V_{10}O_{28}]^{6-}$)
$VOSO_4$	vanadyl sulfate

REFERENCES

1. D. C. Crans, K. Kostenkova, *Commun. Chem.* **2020**, *3*, 104.
2. C. Van Cleave, D.C. Crans, *Inorganics*, **2019**, *7*, 111.
3. J. C. Pessoa, S. Etcheverry, D. Gambino, *Coord. Chem. Rev.* **2015**, *301-302*, 24–48.
4. A. A. Sharfalddin, I. M. Al-Younis, H. A. Mohammed, M. Dhahri, F. Mouffouk, H. Abu Ali, M. J. Anwar, K. A. Qureshi, M. A. Hussien, M. Alghrably, M. Jaremko, N. Alasmael, J. I. Lachowicz, A.-H. Emwas, *Inorganics*, **2022**, *10*, 244.
5. S. Treviño, A. Díaz, E. Sánchez-Lara, B. L. Sanchez-Gaytan, J. M. Perez-Aguilar, E. González-Vergara, *Biol. Trace Elem. Res.* **2019**, *188*, 68–98.
6. L. Gourdon, K. Cariou, G. Gasser, *Chem. Soc. Rev.* **2022**, *51*, 1167–1195.
7. K. H. Thompson, J. Lichter, C. LeBel, M. C. Scaife, J. H. McNeill, C. Orvig, *J. Inorg. Biochem.* **2009**, *103*, 554–558.
8. D. Rehder, *Future Med. Chem.* **2012**, *4*, 1823–1837.
9. G. Scalese, K. Kostenkova, D. C. Crans, D. Gambino, *Curr. Opin. Chem. Biol.* **2022**, *67*, 102127.
10. J. A. Drewry, P. T. Gunning, *Coord. Chem. Rev.* **2011**, *255*, 459–472.
11. M. Pellei, F. Del Bello, M. Porchia, C. Santini, *Coord. Chem. Rev.* **2021**, *445*, 214088.
12. R. Hou, Y. He, G. Yan, S. Hou, Z. Xie, C. Liao, *Eur. J. Med. Chem.* **2021**, *226*, 113877.
13. D. C. Crans, M. Mahroof-Tahir, M. D. Johnson, P. C. Wilkins, L. Yang, K. Robbins, A. Johnson, J. A. Alfano, M. E. Godzala, L. T. Austin, G. R. Willsky, *Inorg. Chim. Acta.* **2003**, *356*, 365–378.
14. K. H. Thompson, C. Orvig, *J. Inorg. Biochem.* **2006**, *100*, 1925–1935.
15. G. R. Willsky, L.-H. Chi, M. Godzala, P. J. Kostyniak, J. J. Smee, A. M. Trujillo, J. A. Alfano, W. Ding, Z. Hu, D. C. Crans, *Coord. Chem. Rev.* **2011**, *255*, 2258–2269.
16. H. Sakurai, *The Chemical Record.* **2002**, *2*, pp. 237–248.
17. M. Aureliano, A. L. D. Sousa-Coelho, C. C. Dolan, D. A. Roess, D. C. Crans, *Int. J. Mol. Sci.* **2023**, *24*, 5382.
18. D. C. Crans, L. Yang, A. Haase, X. Yang, in *Metallo-Drugs: Development and Action of Anticancer Agents*, Eds.: A. Sigel, H. Sigel, E. Freisinger, R. K. O. Sigel, De Gruyter, Berlin, Boston, **2018**, pp. 251–280.
19. M. Aureliano, N. I. Gumerova, G. Sciortino, E. Garribba, A. Rompel, D. C. Crans, *Coord. Chem. Rev.* **2021**, *447*, 214143.
20. T. Scior, A. J. Guevara-Garcia, Q.-T. Do, P. Bernard, S. Laufer, *Curr. Med. Chem.* **2016**, *23*, 2874–2891.
21. D. C. Crans, *J. Org. Chem.* **2015**, *80*, 11899–11915.

22. T. Scior, H. H. Abdallah, S. F. Z. Mustafa, J. A. Guevara-García, D. Rehder, *Inorg. Chim. Acta.* **2021**, *519*, 120287.
23. K. Kostenkova, G. Scalese, D. Gambino, D. C. Crans, *Curr. Opin. Chem. Biol.* **2022**, *69*, 102155.
24. J. Costa Pessoa, I. Tomaz, *Curr. Med. Chem.* **2010**, *17*, 3701–3738.
25. D. C. Crans, J. J. Smee, E. Gaidamauskas, L. Yang, *Chem. Rev.* **2004**, *104*, 849–902.
26. N. D. Chasteen, *Struct. Bonding*, **1983**, *53*, 107–138.
27. M. Valko, H. Morris, T. D. M. Cronin, *Curr. Med. Chem.* **2005**, *12*, 1161–1208.
28. M. Valko, C.J. Rhodes, J. Moncol, M. Izakovic, M. Mazur, *Chem.-Biol. Interact.* **2006**, *160*, 1–40.
29. D. C. Crans, B. J. Peters, X. Wu, C. C. McLauchlan, *Coord. Chem. Rev.* **2017**, *344*, 115–130.
30. J. C. Pessoa, M. F. A. Santos, I. Correia, D. Sanna, G. Sciortino, E. Garriba, *Coord. Chem. Rev.* **2021**, *449*, 214192.
31. S. Semiz, *J. Trace Elem. Med. Biol.* **2022**, *69*, 126887.
32. P. W. Winter, A. Al-Qatati, A. L. Wolf-Ringwall, S. Schoeberl, P. B. Chatterjee, B. G. Barisas, D. A. Roess, D. C. Crans, *Dalton Trans.* **2012**, *41*, 6419–6430.
33. A. Al-Quatati, F. L. Fontes, G. B. Barisas, D. Zhang, D. A. Roess, D. C. Crans, *Dalton Trans.* **2013**, *42*, 11912–11920
34. D. Althumairy, H. A. Murakami, D. Zhang, B. G. Barisas, D. A. Roess, D. C. Crans, *J. Inorg. Biochem.* **2020**, *203*, 110873.
35. D. Althumairy, K. Postal, B. G. Barisas, G. G. Nunes, D. A. Roess, D. C. Crans, *Metallomics*, **2020**, *12*, 1044–1061.
36. N. Samart, D. Althumairy, D. Zhang, D. A. Roess, D. C. Crans, *Coord. Chem. Rev.* **2020**, *416*, 213286.
37. K. Kostenkova, D. Althumairy, A. Rajan, U. Kortz, B. G. Barisas, D. A. Roess, D. C. Crans, *Front. Chem. Biol.* **2023**, *2*, 1126975.
38. V. A. Ferretti, I. E. León, *Inorganics*, **2022**, *10*, 47.
39. A. Levina, D. C. Crans, P. A. Lay, *Coord. Chem. Rev.* **2017**, *352*, 473–498.
40. D. C. Crans, K. A. Woll, K. Prusinskas, M. D. Johnson, E. Norkus, *Inorg. Chem.* **2013**, *52*, 12262–12275.
41. N. Samart, Z. Arhouma, S. Kumar, H. A. Murakami, D. C. Crick, D. C. Crans, *Front. Chem.* **2018**, *6*. https://www.frontiersin.org/articles/10.3389/fchem.2018.00519/full
42. M. Aureliano, D. C. Crans, *J. Inorg. Biochem.* **2009**, *103*, 536–546.
43. M. Aureliano, N. I. Gumerova, G. Sciortino, E. Garriba, C. C. McLauchlan, A. Rompel, D. C. Crans, *Coord. Chem. Rev.* **2022**, *454*, 214344.
44. G. R. Willsky, K. Halvorsen, M. E. Godzala Iii, L.-H. Chi, M. J. Most, P. Kaszynski, D. C. Crans, A. B. Goldfine, P. J. Kostyniak, *Metallomics*, **2013**, *5*, 1491–1502.
45. J. Kamta, M. Chaar, A. Ande, D. A. Altomare, S. Ait-Oudhia, *Front. Oncol.* **2017**, *7*. https://www.frontiersin.org/journals/oncology/articles/10.3389/fonc.2017.00064/full
46. C. A. Shaw, D. Li, L. Tomljenovic, *Immunotherapy*, **2014**, *6*, 1055–1071.
47. J. Kieler, A. Gromek, N. I. Nissen, *Acta Chir. Scand. Suppl.* **1965**, *343*, 154–164.
48. P. Köpf-Maier, H. Köpf, *Drugs Future*, **1986**, *11*, 297–319.
49. S. Mahanty, D. Raghav, K. Rathinasamy, *J. Biol. Inorg. Chem.* **2021**, *26*, 511–531.
50. M. C. Vlasiou, K. S. Pafiti, *Anti-Cancer Agents Med. Chem.* **2021**, *21*, 2111–2116.
51. E. Kioseoglou, S. Petanidis, C. Gabriel, A. Salifoglou, *Coord. Chem. Rev.* **2015**, *301-302*, 87–105.
52. O. J. D'Cruz, F. M. Uckun, *Expert Opin. Invest. Drugs*, **2002**, *11*, 1829–1836.
53. P. Nunes, I. Correia, I. Cavaco, F. Marques, T. Pinheiro, F. Avecilla, J. C. Pessoa, *J. Inorg. Biochem.* **2021**, *217*, 111350.

54. M. L. Cacicedo, M. C. Ruiz, S. Scioli-Montoto, M. E. Ruiz, M. A. Fernández, R. M. Torres-Sanchez, E. J. Baran, G. R. Castro, I. E. León, *New J. Chem.* **2019**, *43*, 17726–17734.

55. I. E. León, P. Díez, S. B. Etcheverry, M. Fuentes, *Metallomics*, **2016**, *8*, 739–749.

56. S. Roy, S. Mallick, T. Chakraborty, N. Ghosh, A. K. Singh, S. Manna, S. Majumdar, *Food Chem.* **2015**, *173*, 1172–1178.

57. S. B. Etcheverry, E. G. Ferrer, L. Naso, J. Rivadeneira, V. Salinas, P. A. M. Williams, JBIC, *J. Biol. Inorg. Chem.* **2008**, *13*, 435–447.

58. E. G. Ferrer, M. V. Salinas, M. J. Correa, L. Naso, D. A. Barrio, S. B. Etcheverry, L. Lezama, T. Rojo, P. A. M. Williams, JBIC, *J. Biol. Inorg. Chem.* **2006**, *11*, 791–801.

59. S. Selvaraj, U. M. Krishnan, *J. Med. Chem.* **2021**, *64*, 12435–12452.

60. M. S. Islas, L. G. Naso, L. Lezama, M. Valcarcel, C. Salado, M. Roura-Ferrer, E. G. Ferrer, P. A. M. Williams, *J. Inorg. Biochem.* **2015**, *149*, 12–24.

61. J. J. Martínez Medina, L. G. Naso, A. L. Pérez, A. Rizzi, N. B. Okulik, E. G. Ferrer, P. A. M. Williams, *J. Photochem. Photobiol., A*, **2017**, *344*, 84–100.

62. L. G. Naso, L. Lezama, T. Rojo, S. B. Etcheverry, M. Valcarcel, M. Roura, C. Salado, E. G. Ferrer, P. A. M. Williams, *Chem.-Biol. Interact.* **2013**, *206*, 289–301.

63. L. Naso, V. R. Martínez, L. Lezama, C. Salado, M. Valcarcel, E. G. Ferrer, P. A. M. Williams, *Bioorg. Med. Chem. Lett.* **2016**, *24*, 4108–4119.

64. S. Roy, S. Majumdar, A. K. Singh, B. Ghosh, N. Ghosh, S. Manna, T. Chakraborty, S. Mallick, *Biol. Trace Elem. Res.* **2015**, *166*, 183–200.

65. I. E. Leon, A. L. Di Virgilio, V. Porro, C. I. Muglia, L. G. Naso, P. A. M. Williams, M. Bollati-Fogolin, S. B. Etcheverry, *Dalton Trans.* **2013**, *42*, 11868–11880.

66. P. K. Sasmal, A. K. Patra, M. Nethaji, A. R. Chakravarty, *Inorg. Chem.* **2007**, *46*, 11112–11121.

67. B. Balaji, B. Balakrishnan, S. Perumalla, A. A. Karande, A. R. Chakravarty, *Eur. J. Med. Chem.* **2014**, *85*, 458–467.

68. B. Banik, K. Somyajit, G. Nagaraju, A. R. Chakravarty, *Dalton Trans.* **2014**, *43*, 13358–13369.

69. A. Kumar, A. Dixit, S. Sahoo, S. Banerjee, A. Bhattacharyya, A. Garai, A. A. Karande, A. R. Chakravarty, *J. Inorg. Biochem.* **2020**, *202*, 110817.

70. A. Kumar, A. Dixit, S. Banerjee, A. Bhattacharyya, A. Garai, A. A. Karande, A. R. Chakravarty, *Med. Chem. Comm.* **2016**, *7*, 1398–1404.

71. L. Noriega, M. E. Castro, J. M. Perez-Aguilar, N. A. Caballero, B. L. Sanchez-Gaytan, E. González-Vergara, F. J. Melendez, *J. Inorg. Biochem.* **2020**, *203*, 110862.

72. B. Sanasam, M. K. Raza, D. Musib, M. Pal, M. Pal, M. Roy, *ChemistrySelect*, **2020**, *5*, 13824–13830.

73. Y. Nie, W. Zhang, W. Xiao, W. Zeng, T. Chen, W. Huang, X. Wu, Y. Kang, J. Dong, W. Luo, X. Ji, *Biomaterials*, **2022**, *289*, 121791.

74. A. Levina, D. C. Crans, P. A. Lay, *Pharmaceutics*, **2022**, *14*, 790.

75. L. Hernández, M. L. Araujo, W. Madden, E. Del Carpio, V. Lubes, G. Lubes, *J. Inorg. Biochem.* **2022**, *229*, 111712.

76. M. Kongot, N. Dohare, D. S. Reddy, N. Pereira, R. Patel, M. Subramanian, A. Kumar, *J. Trace Elem. Med. Biol.* **2019**, *51*, 176–190.

77. P. Mokhtari, G. Mohammadnezhad, *Polyhedron*, **2022**, *215*, 115655.

78. S. S. Hassan, E. A. Bedir, A. E.-R. M. Hamza, A. M. Ahmed, N. M. Ibrahim, M. S. Abd El-Ghany, N. N. Khattab, B. M. Emeira, M. M. Salama, E. F. Mohamed, D. B. Fayed, *Appl. Organomet. Chem.* **2022**, *36*, e6804.

79. M. R. Rodríguez, L. M. Balsa, J. Del Plá, J. García-Tojal, R. Pis-Diez, B. S. Parajón-Costa, I. E. León, A. C. González-Baró, *New J. Chem.* **2019**, *43*, 11784–11794.

80. Y. Bai, H. Zhang, Y. Wang, L. Zhu, T. Shi, H. Wei, J. Xiao, Y. Zhang, Z. Wang, *Front. Pharmacol.* **2021**, *11*. https://www.frontiersin.org/journals/pharmacology/articles/10.3389/fphar.2020.596525/full

81. G. Sahu, E. R. T. Tiekink, R. Dinda, *Inorganics*, **2021**, *9*, 66.

82. N. Ribeiro, A. M. Galvão, C. S. B. Gomes, H. Ramos, R. Pinheiro, L. Saraiva, E. Ntungwe, V. Isca, P. Rijo, I. Cavaco, F. Ramilo-Gomes, R. C. Guedes, J. C. Pessoa, I. Correia, *New J. Chem.* **2019**, *43*, 17801–17818.

83. H. A. Rudbari, A. Saadati, M. Aryaeifar, I. Correia, F. Marques, O. Blacque, N. Micale, *Bioorg. Med. Chem. Lett.*, *49*, 128285.

84. G. Sahu, S. A. Patra, P. D. Pattanayak, W. Kaminsky, R. Dinda, *Inorg. Chem.* **2023**, *62*, 6722–6739.

85. D. C. Crans, J. T. Koehn, S. M. Petry, C. M. Glover, A. Wijetunga, R. Kaur, A. Levina, P. A. Lay, *Dalton Trans.* **2019**, *48*, 6383–6395.

86. A. Levina, A. Pires Vieira, A. Wijetunga, R. Kaur, J. T. Koehn, D. C. Crans, P. A. Lay, *Angew. Chem., Int. Ed.* **2020**, *59*, 15834–15838.

87. H. A. Murakami, C. Uslan, A. A. Haase, J. T. Koehn, A. P. Vieira, D. J. Gaebler, J. Hagan, C. N. Beuning, N. Proschogo, A. Levina, P. A. Lay, D. C. Crans, *Inorg. Chem.* **2022**, *61*, 20757–20773.

88. B. K. Biswas, N. Biswas, S. Saha, A. Rahaman, D. P. Mandal, S. Bhattacharjee, N. Sepay, E. Zangrando, E. Garribba, C. Roy Choudhury, *J. Inorg. Biochem.* **2022**, *237*, 111980.

89. D. Crans, L. Yang, T. Jakusch, T. Kiss, *Inorg. Chem.* **2000**, *39*, 4409–4416.

90. A. Bergeron, K. Kostenkova, M. Selman, H. A. Murakami, E. Owens, N. Haribabu, R. Arulanandam, J.-S. Diallo, D. C. Crans, *BioMetals*, **2019**, *32*, 545–561.

91. T. M. McAusland, J. P. van Vloten, L. A. Santry, M. M. Guilleman, A. D. Rghei, E. M. Ferreira, J. C. Ingrao, R. Arulanandam, P. P. Major, L. Susta, K. Karimi, J.-S. Diallo, B. W. Bridle, S. K. Wootton, *Mol. Ther.--Oncolytics*, **2021**, *20*, 306–324.

92. J.-S. Diallo, D.C. Crans, R. Arulanandam, Canada, United States, 2022. International Application Published under the Patent Cooperation Treaty (PCT). International Publication Data 10 November 2022 (10.11.2022); International publication number WO 2022/232944 A1.

93. B. Wong, A. Bergeron, A. Alluqmani, G. Maznyi, A. Chen, R. Arulanandam, J.-S. Diallo, *Mol. Ther. - Oncolytics*, **2022**, *25*, 146–159.

94. L.-P. Lu, J.-H. Liu, S.-H. Cen, Y.-L. Jiang, G.-Q. Hu, *Bioorg. Med. Chem. Lett.* **2019**, *29*, 681–683.

95. L.-P. Lu, F.-Z. Suo, Y.-L. Feng, L.-L. Song, Y. Li, Y.-J. Li, K.-T. Wang, *Eur. J. Med. Chem.* **2019**, *176*, 1–10.

96. D. C. Crans, L. Henry, G. Cardiff, B. I. Posner, in *Essential Metals in Medicine: Therapeutic Use and Toxicity of Metal Ions in the Clinic*, Guest-Ed.: P. L. Carver, Eds A. Sigel, E. Freisinger, R. K. O. Sigel, De Gruyter, Berlin, Boston, **2019**, pp. 203–230.

97. Y. Tian, H. Qi, G. Wang, L. Li, D. Zhou, *BioMetals*, **2021**, *34*, 557–571.

98. J.-X. Wu, Y.-H. Hong, X.-G. Yang, JBIC, *J. Biol. Inorg. Chem.* **2016**, *21*, 919–929.

99. M. Selman, C. Rousso, A. Bergeron, H. H. Son, R. Krishnan, N. A. El-Sayes, O. Varette, A. Chen, F. Le Boeuf, F. Tzelepis, J. C. Bell, D. C. Crans, J.-S. Diallo, *Mol. Ther.* **2018**, *26*, 56–69.

100. G. G. Nunes, A. C. Bonatto, C. G. de Albuquerque, A. Barison, R. R. Ribeiro, D. F. Back, A. V. C. Andrade, E. L. de Sá, F. d. O. Pedrosa, J. F. Soares, E. M. de Souza, *J. Inorg. Biochem.* **2012**, *108*, 36–46.

101. Y.-T. Li, C.-Y. Zhu, Z.-Y. Wu, M. Jiang, C.-W. Yan, *Transition Metal Chem.* **2010**, *35*, 597–603.

102. M. S. Alqahtani, M. Kazi, M. A. Alsenaidy, M. Z. Ahmad, *Front. Pharmacol.* **2021**, *12.* https://www.frontiersin.org/journals/pharmacology/articles/10.3389/fphar.2021.618411/full

103. S. S. Hallan, J. Amirian, A. Brangule, D. Bandere, *Nanomaterials*, **2022**, *12*, 1146.

104. T. Boztepe, S. Scioli-Montoto, M. E. Ruiz, V. A. Alvarez, G. R. Castro, I. E. León, *New J. Chem.* **2021**, *45*, 821–830.

105. Y. Gou, G. Huang, J. Li, F. Yang, H. Liang, *Coord. Chem. Rev.* **2021**, *441*, 213975.

106. R. S. D'Amico, M. K. Aghi, M. A. Vogelbaum, J. N. Bruce, *J. Neuro-Oncol.* **2021**, *151*, 415–427.

107. C. D. Nwagwu, A. V. Immidisetti, M. Y. Jiang, O. Adeagbo, D. C. Adamson, A.-M. Carbonell, *Pharmaceutics*, **2021**, *13*, 561.

108. J. H. Kang, A. Desjardins, *Neuro-Oncol. Pract.* **2021**, *9*, 24–34.

109. M. Alyami, M. Hübner, F. Grass, N. Bakrin, L. Villeneuve, N. Laplace, G. Passot, O. Glehen, V. Kepenekian, *Lancet Oncol.* **2019**, *20*, e368–e377.

110. L. A. W. de Jong, N. P. van Erp, L. Bijelic, *Clin. Cancer Res.* **2021**, *27*, 1830–1832.

111. D. Hu, H. Xu, W. Zhang, X. Xu, B. Xiao, X. Shi, Z. Zhou, N. K. H. Slater, Y. Shen, *J. Tang, Biomater.* **2021**, *277*, 121130.

112. N. A. ElSayed, G. Aleppo, V. R. Aroda, R. R. Bannuru, F. M. Brown, D. Bruemmer, B. S. Collins, M. E. Hilliard, D. Isaacs, E. L. Johnson, S. Kahan, K. Khunti, J. Leon, S. K. Lyons, M. L. Perry, P. Prahalad, R. E. Pratley, J. J. Seley, R. C. Stanton, R. A. Gabbay, American Diabetes Association. *Diabetes Care*, **2022**, *46*, S19–S40.

113. J. L. Domingo, M. Gómez, *Food Chem. Toxicol.*, **2016**, *95*, 137–141.

114. S. Treviño, D. Velázquez-Vázquez, E. Sánchez-Lara, A. Diaz-Fonseca, J. Á. Flores-Hernandez, A. Pérez-Benítez, E. Brambila-Colombres, E. González-Vergara, *Med. Cell. Longevity*, **2016**, *2016*, 6058705.

115. S. Treviño, E. González-Vergara, *New J. Chem.* **2019**, *43*, 17850–17862.

116. E. Sánchez-Lara, S. Treviño, B. L. Sánchez-Gaytán, E. Sánchez-Mora, M. Eugenia Castro, F. J. Meléndez-Bustamante, M. A. Méndez-Rojas, E. González-Vergara, *Front. Chem.* **2018**, *6*.

117. O. I. Alajrawy, S. F. Tuleab, E. T. Alshammary, *J. Mol. Struct.* **2022**, *1269*, 133821.

118. A. Shaik, V. Kondaparthy, R. Aveli, L. Vemulapalli, D. D. Manwal, *Appl. Organomet. Chem.* **2022**, *36*, e6710.

119. L. M. A. Lima, H. Murakami, D. J. Gaebler, W. E. Silva, M. F. Belian, E. C. Lira, D. C. Crans, *Inorganics*, **2021**, *9*, 42.

120. L. M. A. Lima, A. K. J. P. F. da Silva, E. K. Batista, K. Postal, K. Kostenkova, A. Fenton, D. C. Crans, W. E. Silva, M. F. Belian, E. C. Lira, *J. Inorg. Bioch.* **2023**, *241*, 112127.

121. A. Ceriello, L. Quagliaro, B. Catone, R. Pascon, M. Piazzola, B. Bais, G. Marra, L. Tonutti, C. Taboga, E. Motz, *Diabetes Care*, **2002**, *25*, 1439–1443.

122. A. Likidlilid, N. Patchanans, T. Peerapatdit, C. Sriratanasathavorn, *J. Med. Assoc. Thai.* **2010**, *93*, 682–693.

123. G. Davì, A. Falco, C. Patrono, *Antioxid. Redox Signal.* **2005**, *7*, 256–268.

124. F. Giacco, M. Brownlee, *Circ. Res.* **2010**, *107*, 1058–1070.

125. A. de Souza Bastos, D. T. Graves, A. P. de Melo Loureiro, C. R. Júnior, S. C. T. Corbi, F. Frizzera, R. M. Scarel-Caminaga, N. O. Câmara, O. M. Andriankaja, M. I. Hiyane, S. R. P. Orrico, *J. Diabetes Complications*, **2016**, *30*, 1593–1599.

126. E. Rendra, V. Riabov, D. M. Mossel, T. Sevastyanova, M. C. Harmsen, J. Kzhyshkowska, *Immunobiology*, **2019**, *224*, 242–253.

127. R. Yanardag, S. Tunali, Mol. *Cell. Biochem.* **2006**, *286*, 153–159.

128. D. A. Rusanov, J. Zou, M. V. Babak, *Pharmaceuticals*, **2022**, *15*, 453.

129. M. S. Bhuiyan, K. Fukunaga, *J. Pharmacol. Sci.* **2009**, *110*, 1–13.

130. D. C. Crans, M. L. Tarlton, C. C. McLauchlan, *Eur. J. Inorg. Chem.* **2014**, *2014*, 4450–4468.

131. C. C. McLauchlan, B. J. Peters, G. R. Willsky, D. C. Crans, *Coord. Chem. Rev.* **2015**, *301-302*, 163–199.

132. B. Feng, Y. Dong, B. Shang, B. Zhang, D. C. Crans, X. Yang, *Adv. Funct. Mater.* **2022**, *32*, 2108645.

133. S. K. Panchal, S. Wanyonyi, L. Brown, *Curr. Hypertens. Rep.* **2017**, *19*, 10.

134. D. C. Crans, *J. Inorg. Biochem.* **2000**, *80*, 123–131.

135. M. Z. Mehdi, A. K. Srivastava, *Arch. Biochem. Biophys.* **2005**, *440*, 158–164.

136. D. Rehder, in *Interrelations between Essential Metal Ions and Human Diseases*, Eds.: A. Sigel, H. Sigel, R. K. O. Sigel, Springer, Dordrecht, The Netherlands, **2013**, pp. 139–169.

137. K. T. Keyes, J. Xu, B. Long, C. Zhang, Z. Hu, Y. Ye, *Am. J. Physiol.: Heart Circ. Physiol.* **2010**, *298*, H1198–H1208.

138. R. M. C. Gândara, S. S. Soares, H. Martins, C. Gutiérrez-Merino, M. Aureliano, *J. Inorg. Biochem.* **2005**, *99*, 1238–1244.

139. S. S. Soares, H. Martins, R. O. Duarte, J. J. G. Moura, J. Coucelo, C. Gutiérrez-Merino, M. Aureliano, *J. Inorg. Biochem.* **2007**, *101*, 80–88.

140. K. H. Cheeseman, *Mol. Aspects Med.* **1993**, *14*, 191–197.

141. Z. Zhang, S. S. Leonard, C. Huang, V. Vallyathan, V. Castranova, X. Shi, *Free Radical Biol. Med.* **2003**, *34*, 1333–1342.

142. L. S. Capella, M. R. Gefé, E. F. Silva, O. Affonso-Mitidieri, A. G. Lopes, V. M. Rumjanek, M. A. M. Capella, *Arch. Biochem. Biophys.* **2002**, *406*, 65–72.

143. X.-G. Yang, X.-D. Yang, L. Yuan, K. Wang, D. C. Crans, *Pharm. Res.* **2004**, *21*, 1026–1033.

144. D. Lapenna, G. Ciofani, S. D. Pierdomenico, M. A. Giamberardino, F. Cuccurullo, *Free Radical Biol. Med.* **2001**, *31*, 331–335.

145. O. V. Taso, A. Philippou, A. Moustogiannis, E. Zevolis, M. Koutsilieris, *Ann. Res. Hosp.* **2019**, *3*. https://arh.amegroups.org/article/view/4663/pdf

146. I. Dalle-Donne, R. Rossi, R. Colombo, D. Giustarini, A. Milzani, *Clin. Chem.* **2006**, *52*, 601–623.

147. X. L. Shi, N. S. Dalal, *Arch. Biochem. Biophys.* **1993**, *307*, 336–341.

148. F. A. Al-Salmi, R. Z. Hamza, *Curr. Issues Mol. Biol.* **2022**, *44*, 94–104.

149. F. Ghalichi, A. Ostadrahimi, M. Saghafi-Asl, *J. Trace Elem. Med. Biol.* **2022**, *71*, 126955.

150. L. Ji, D. Hu, C. Pan, J. Weng, Y. Huo, C. Ma, Y. Mu, C. Hao, Q. Ji, X. Ran, B. Su, H. Zhuo, K. A. Fox, M. Weber, D. Zhang, *Am. J. Med.* **2013**, *126*, 925.e911-922.

151. A. Wilk, B. Wiszniewska, D. Szypulska-Koziarska, P. Kaczmarek, M. Romanowski, J. Różański, M. Słojewski, K. Ciechanowski, M. Marchelek-Myśliwiec, E. Kalisińska, *Biol. Trace Elem. Res.* **2017**, *180*, 1–5.

152. X.-C. Liu, E. Strodl, L.-H. Huang, B.-J. Hu, W.-Q. Chen, *Atmosphere*, **2022**, *13*. Doi:10.3390/atmos13122022. https://www.mdpi.com/2073-4433/13/12/2022

153. F.L.Assem, A.Oskarsson, **2015**, https://www.sciencedirect.com/topics/pharmacology-toxicology-and-pharmaceutical-science/vanadium-compounds

154. G. Scalese, Z. Arhouma, K. Kostenkova, L. Pérez-Díaz, D.C. Crick, D. Gambino, D.C. Crans, *J. Inorg. Biochem.* **2022**, *237*, 111984.

155. D. C. Crans, K. Postal, J. A. MacGregor, *Metal Toxicology Handbook*, CRC Press, Boca Raton, **2020**, p. 14, Chapter 6.

3 Ruthenium-Phthalocyanine Compounds as Prototypes for Photodynamic Therapy

Amanda Blanque Becceneri,
Matheus Torelli Martin, and Francisco Rinaldi Neto
Faculty of Pharmaceutical Sciences of Ribeirão Preto
Universidade de São Paulo
Ribeirão Preto – SP, 14040-903, Brazil

Peter C. Ford
Department of Chemistry and Biochemistry
University of California, Santa Barbara
Santa Barbara, California 93110-9510, USA

Roberto Santana da Silva
Faculty of Pharmaceutical Sciences of Ribeirão Preto
Universidade de São Paulo
Ribeirão Preto – SP, 14040-903, Brazil
Department of Chemistry and Biochemistry
University of California, Santa Barbara
Santa Barbara, California 93110-9510, USA

CONTENTS

DOI: 10.1201/9781003361756-3

ABSTRACT

Cancer is one of the leading causes of death worldwide. Contemporary therapies do
not achieve the expected effectiveness, the treatment is often non-selective, and its
application is associated with several significant side effects, reducing the quality of
life of patients who underwent surgery and their long and expensive hospitalization.
Photodynamic therapy appears as a suitable clinical treatment once it is a non-invasive
technique and uses a photosensitizer, oxygen, and light irradiation to kill cancer cells.
Perhaps the main limitation of PDT is oxygen, once the tumor is mainly hypoxic. In
this chapter, we propose the use of ruthenium-phthalocyanine compounds in anticancer therapy, essentially using the basic principles of photodynamic therapy. The evaluation of photocytotoxic effects is described as a function of the structure-activity
relationship as well as the synergistic effect between nitric oxide and reactive oxygen
species generated by light irradiation in the therapeutic window.

KEYWORDS

Ruthenium; phthalocyanine; photodynamic therapy; nitric oxide; reactive
oxygen species

1   INTRODUCTION

Photodynamic therapy (PDT) is a selective and non-invasive technique that has
been highlighted in the treatment of cancer when compared to traditional therapies
such as chemotherapy [1,2]. This technique consists of using a photosensitizer (PS),
which is activated by visible light irradiation [3]. The deactivation of the excited PS
can occur by energy transfer to oxygen-generating reactive oxygen species (ROS),
such as singlet oxygen, by emission of light (fluorescence or phosphorescence), or
by non-radiative deactivation to release its energy as heat (Figure 1).

The action of free radicals, which are highly reactive, can damage the local
vasculature, generate an inflammatory response, and trigger cell death via apoptosis and/or necrosis [3–8]. PDT is already approved by the American regulatory

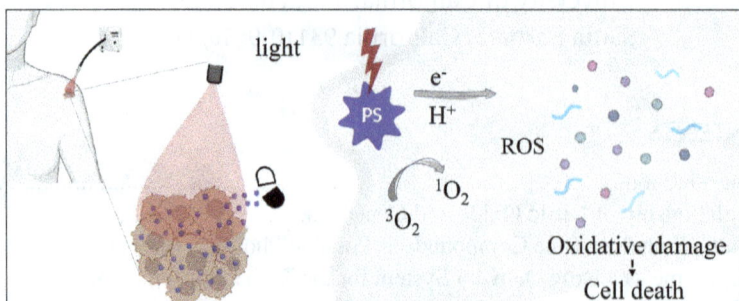

FIGURE 1   Schematic diagram illustrating the mechanistic action of the activated
photosensitizing system.

agency, the Food and Drug Administration, and has advantages in the treatment of cancer, such as few adverse effects on patients, impairment of the vasculature close to the tumor, and the possibility of accurately limiting the region receiving treatment. This clinical process can be associated with other types of treatments since it is less subject to cross-resistance with drugs already used and there is no impediment if it is necessary to use other therapies later [3,5,9,10]. The PS agents can have a natural origin or be produced synthetically in laboratories [4]. The most exploited organic PSs are tetrapyrrolic derivatives composed of porphyrin or chlorin chromophores. The first photosensitizer approved by the Food and Drug Administration was the oligomer derived from porphyrin, commercially known as Photofrin®, in 1993. This is still the most popular and is used in the treatment of different types of tumors, such as liver, bladder, and brain. Some PSs, such as Photofrin®, have limitations, such as absorption outside the therapeutic window, or are less effective at penetration into targeted sites in the body due to tissue spreading and absorption processes. They also demonstrate skin photosensitivity reactions [2,4,9,11,12]. Therefore, alternative PSs would be desirable. An ideal PS has to present specific characteristics, such as not being toxic until photoactivated and preferential accumulation in tumor cells, which allows greater accuracy in the treatment [3–6]. Phthalocyanine dyes represent a type of PS that has been explored recently. These are fluorescent aromatic compounds displaying strong absorptions at wavelengths that facilitate tissue penetration [13]. A number of metal complexes also have characteristics that make them potential PS agents for use in PDT (Table 1). Among these desired characteristics is the range of oxidation states, which allows for various types of bonds and different electronic configurations [2]. The potential for the clinical application of metal-based PSs for cancer treatment could be evidenced by the entry of the ruthenium-based photosensitizer TLD-1433 into clinical trials for bladder cancer and also the approval for clinical use in some countries of the palladium-based photosensitizer TOOKAD® for the treatment of prostate cancer (Figure 2) [14].

Table 1 provides an overview of the effects of various metal-based complexes on different types of cancer cells, both under light irradiation (phototoxicity) and in the absence of light (cytotoxicity).

The expected reactivity of the metal-based compounds can be represented in Figure 3.

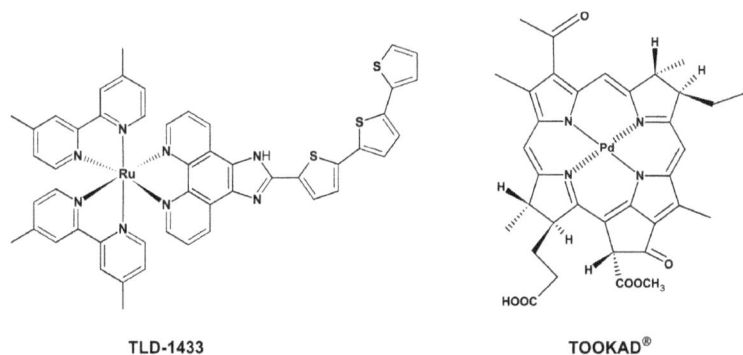

TLD-1433   TOOKAD®

FIGURE 2   Chemical structure of TLD-1433 and TOOKAD®.

TABLE 1
Overview of the Effects of Various Metal-Based Complexes on Different Types of Cancer Cells

Complex	Metal	Cell Lines	Phototoxicity IC_{50} (µM)	Cytotoxicity IC_{50} (µM)	Ref
Pd-Tripor Palladium porphyrin complex	Palladium	Human cervical carcinoma HeLa	9.6	> 30	[15]
[2,10,16,24-tetrakis-(1-sulfide-2-thio-o-carboranyl) phthalocyaninato Zn(II)]	Zinc	Breast cancer MCF-7	74.55	337.82	[16]
[2,10,16,24-tetrakis-(1-sulfide-2-thio-o-carboranyl) phthalocyaninato Co(II)]	Cobalt	Breast cancer MCF-7	81.55	90.04	[16]
{Ir[(2-(2,2′:6′,2″-terpyridin-4′-yl) porphyrin]$_2$}(PF$_6^{.}$)$_3$	Iridium	Melanoma B16-F10	1.34	> 10	[17]
Picolylamine-functionalized porphyrin zinc complex	Zinc	Breast Cancer MDA-MB-231	7	> 100000	[18]
5,10,15,20-tetra[4-methoxy-3-(1,4,7,10-tetraoxoundecyl)phenyl] porphyrin zinc(II)	Zinc	Bladder cancer 5637	0.01556	> 0.0250	[19]
5,10,15,20-tetra[3-methoxy-4-(1,4,7,10-tetraoxoundecyl)phenyl] porphyrin zinc(II)	Zinc	Prostate carcinoma LNCaP	0.04863	> 0.0250	[19]
[Ru(bpy)$_2$(3-Py)TMPPCl]Cl o	Ruthenium	Lung cancer A549	54.2	> 500	[20]
[Ru(bpy)$_2$(3-Py)TMPPCl]Cl o	Ruthenium	Breast cancer MCF-7	42.3	> 500	[20]
[Ru(phen)$_2$(3-Py)TMPPCl]Cl	Ruthenium	Lung cancer A549	39.7	> 500	[20]
[Ru(phen)$_2$(3-Py)TMPPCl]Cl	Ruthenium	Breast cancer MCF-7	52.2	> 500	[20]
[Ru(dmb)$_2$(HMNPIP)](PF$_6$)$_2$	Ruthenium	Lung cancer A549	4	> 200	[21]
[Ru(dmb)$_2$(HMNPIP)](PF$_6$)$_2$	Ruthenium	Breast cancer MCF-7	34.9	> 200	[21]
[Ru(dmb)$_2$(HMNPIP)](PF$_6$)$_2$	Ruthenium	Gastric cancer SGC-7901	> 100	> 200	[21]
[Ru(dmb)$_2$(HMNPIP)](PF$_6$)$_2$	Ruthenium	Esophageal carcinoma Eca-109	45.8	> 200	[21]
[Ru(dmb)$_2$(HMNPIP)](PF$_6$)$_2$	Ruthenium	Human cervical carcinoma HeLa	34.2	> 200	[21]
[Ru(dmb)$_2$(HMNPIP)](PF$_6$)$_2$	Ruthenium	Hepatoma Hep-G2	12.5	> 200	[21]

(Continued)

TABLE 1 (*Continued*)
Overview of the Effects of Various Metal-Based Complexes on Different Types of Cancer Cells

Complex	Metal	Cell Lines	Phototoxicity IC_{50} (μM)	Cytotoxicity IC_{50} (μM)	Ref
[Ru(bpy)$_2$(HMNPIP)](PF$_6$)$_2$	Ruthenium	Lung cancer A549	6.8	> 200	[21]
[Ru(bpy)$_2$(HMNPIP)](PF$_6$)$_2$	Ruthenium	Breast cancer MCF-7	> 100	> 200	[21]
[Ru(bpy)$_2$(HMNPIP)](PF$_6$)$_2$	Ruthenium	Gastric cancer SGC-7901	8.7	> 200	[21]
[Ru(bpy)$_2$(HMNPIP)](PF$_6$)$_2$	Ruthenium	Esophageal carcinoma Eca-109	15.1	> 200	[21]
[Ru(bpy)$_2$(HMNPIP)](PF$_6$)$_2$	Ruthenium	Human cervical carcinoma HeLa	13.8	> 200	[21]
[Ru(bpy)$_2$(HMNPIP)](PF$_6$)$_2$	Ruthenium	Hepatoma Hep-G2	14.6	> 200	[21]
[Ru(phen)$_2$(HMNPIP)](PF$_6$)$_2$	Ruthenium	Lung cancer A549	3	> 200	[21]
[Ru(phen)$_2$(HMNPIP)](PF$_6$)$_2$	Ruthenium	Breast cancer MCF-7	21.5	> 200	[21]
[Ru(phen)$_2$(HMNPIP)](PF$_6$)$_2$	Ruthenium	Gastric cancer SGC-7901	4.9	> 200	[21]
[Ru(phen)$_2$(HMNPIP)](PF$_6$)$_2$	Ruthenium	Esophageal carcinoma Eca-109	13.2	> 200	[21]
[Ru(phen)$_2$(HMNPIP)](PF$_6$)$_2$	Ruthenium	Human cervical carcinoma HeLa	8	> 200	[21]
[Ru(phen)$_2$(HMNPIP)](PF$_6$)$_2$	Ruthenium	Hepatoma Hep-G2	13.3	> 200	[21]

Despite the positive results found in the clinical use of PDT, there are still some obstacles to the successful use of this technique. An important barrier to be circumvented is the fact that most tumors have regions with low concentration of oxygen [23], which is essential for the PDT clinical process [2]. With the aim of overcoming this limitation, other molecules that produce different species of oxygen-independent radicals have been studied as alternatives for PDT (Table 2) and have been highlighted as advances in research involving PDT for cancer treatment [10]. In addition, the combination of PDT with other therapies can create a synergistic effect and thus be a good strategy to overcome the previously detached barriers [24]. Perhaps one of the most studied radicals in the synergistic effect of ROS is nitric oxide (NO).

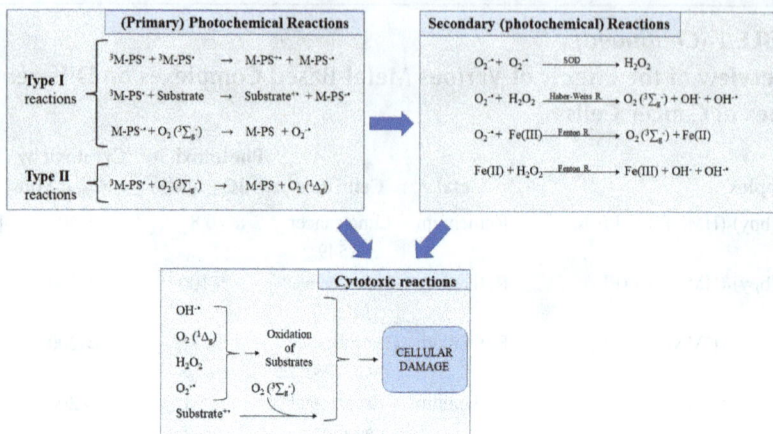

FIGURE 3 Photochemical reactions of ruthenium-photosensitizer (Ru-PS) in the triple excited state (adapted from Ref. [22]).

TABLE 2
Free Radical Generated by Anticancer Compounds Submitted to Light Irradiation

Radicals	Photosensitizer Examples	Mechanism of Action	Ref.
Reactive oxygen species (ROS)	Photofrin, Porfimer Sodium, Verteporfin, Aminolevulinic Acid (ALA), 5-Aminolevulinic Acid Methyl Ester (MAL), Foscan (Temoporfin)	Generate reactive oxygen species upon light activation. Examples of ROS include singlet oxygen ($^1O_2$), superoxide anion ($O_2^{\cdot-}$), and hydroxyl radical ($^\cdot OH$). These ROS induce oxidative stress and cell damage.	[25–36]
Alkoxyl radicals ($RO^\cdot$)	Aluminum Phthalocyanine, Phthalocyanine dyes, Temoporfin (Foscan)	Formed by the reaction of a photosensitizer with molecular oxygen upon light activation. These radicals initiate chain reactions by abstracting hydrogen atoms from cellular components.	[37–42]
Peroxyl radicals ($ROO^\cdot$)	Hypocrellin A, Hypericin	Generated when a photosensitizer reacts with molecular oxygen upon light activation. These radicals propagate chain reactions, causing cellular damage and cell death.	[43–46]
Carbon-centered radicals ($^\cdot CR3$)	Rose Bengal, Hematoporphyrin Derivative (HpD), Chlorin e6	Produced when a photosensitizer molecule absorbs light. These radicals induce oxidative stress by reacting with lipids, proteins, and DNA, resulting in cellular damage and apoptosis.	[47–51]

(Continued)

TABLE 2 (Continued)
Free Radical Generated by Anticancer Compounds Submitted to Light Irradiation

Radicals	Photosensitizer Examples	Mechanism of Action	Ref.
Nitric oxide radicals ($\cdot$NO)	Nitroaniline, Nitroimidazole derivatives, Nitric Oxide-Releasing Porphyrins	Generated by photosensitizers upon light activation. Nitric oxide radicals can act as signaling molecules and exhibit cytotoxic effects when reacting with superoxide anions.	[52–60]
Iodinated Photosensitizers and Iodine radicals ($I\cdot$)	Iodinated Porphyrins, Iodoquinoline derivatives	Iodine radicals can be generated through the homolytic cleavage of an iodine molecule. Iodinated photosensitizers can be used in PDT to generate reactive species, including singlet oxygen and other radicals, upon light activation. These radicals participate in oxidative reactions.	[61–73]
Nitroimidazole derivatives	Misonidazole, Metronidazole, Nimorazole, Etanidazole, Efaproxiral	Nitroimidazole derivatives are a class of compounds that can act with photosensitizers in PDT.	[74–82]

2 RELATIONSHIP OF NITRIC OXIDE AND CANCER

NO is a signaling molecule produced throughout the body, synthesized by the NOS family of enzymes, and well known for participating in different physiological and pathological processes *in vivo* [83–85]. Recently, the role of NO in cancer has been extensively discussed in the literature due to its implications for tumor progression and regression depending on the concentration and exposure time. In some situations, it can act by inducing cell death and, in others, by preserving cells [83,84,86–89]. Although there are already studies demonstrating the effectiveness of NO in the treatment of cancer, research still needs to better explore it due to its variable role depending on its microenvironment [90,91]. The control of the amount of NO in treatments must be very strict, since changes in its levels can lead to disorders [41]. The main strategies for using NO in cancer treatment involve increasing the concentration of this molecule through donor compounds or inhibiting the NOS family of enzymes [92]. High concentrations of NO are known to have antitumor properties, and low concentrations are needed to ensure cell survival [93]. At high concentrations, NO is capable of inducing cell death by apoptosis in different cell types [93]. Based on that, NO donors have been used for the development of new therapies against cancer since they have some advantages, including different mechanisms of NO release and variable half-lives. Interestingly, NO has a high affinity for binding to metals, which makes it possible to use metals as NO donor agents [94].

Recent studies have begun to elucidate the role of NO in different contexts. Non-tumor breast cells grown in 3D culture on Matrigel® form polarized, organized structures called mammary acini, like those found *in vivo*. Tumor mammary cells are not able to form organized structures, so they form clusters of disorganized, non-polarized cells with uncontrolled growth [95]. In a recent study, researchers demonstrated that tumor cells cultured *in vitro* in 2D and 3D and non-tumor breast cells cultured *in vitro* in 2D do not produce NO and increase the expression of some genes that are responsible for disorganizing the functional glandular units. However, these researchers also observed that when adding NO to tumor mammary cells cultured in 3D, the reversal of the malignant phenotype occurred, with the cells being reorganized into organized structures that resemble mammary functional glandular units [96]. Another study demonstrated that mechanical compression forces applied to breast tumor cells lead to the reversal of the malignant phenotype due to increased NO production, as the blockade prevents the reversal [97].

It is important to emphasize that the use of NO also has some limitations, such as cytotoxicity to normal cells and control of the amount of NO in the body, which can trigger effects on the cardiovascular system. However, some NO donors have selectivity for tumor cells, manage to release NO at different times, and can still be combined with other compounds to create a more potent effect [98]. The interest in NO donor agents has grown a lot in the last decade, and the strategy to design compounds capable of releasing NO in a controlled way has constituted one major goal in PDT research [99–104]. The possibility of combining a compound that has multiple actions against cancer is seen as the Holy Grail in PDT (Figure 4). This drove us to explore NO derivative compounds of ruthenium-phthalocyanine and ruthenium-porphyrin as base species for a series of derivative compounds.

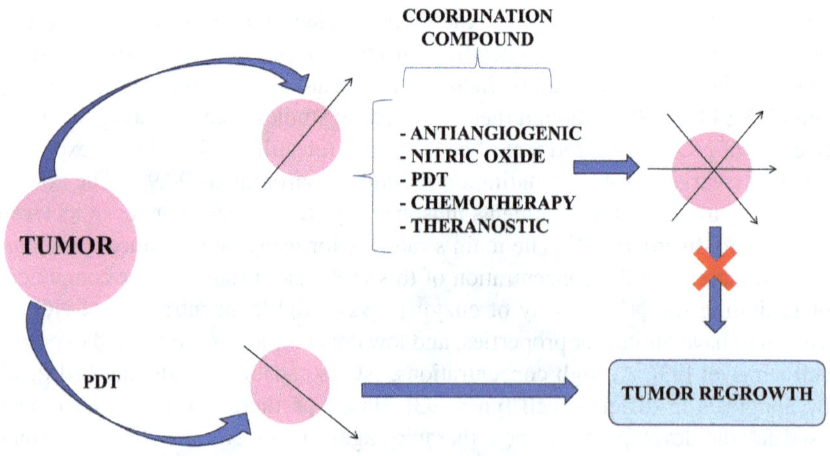

FIGURE 4   Strategy to enhance PDT treatment using metal sensitizers.

3 METAL-PHTHALOCYANINE COMPOUNDS AS POSSIBLE PHOTOSENSITIZERS FOR PDT

Phthalocyanine compounds can be defined as aromatic polycycles with four isoindole units, that is, a benzene ring fused to a pyrrole. The isoindole units are linked through an "aza" bridge. The "aza" bridge is defined as aromatic compounds that have some of the carbon atoms (C) replaced by nitrogen atoms (N). The aromatic rings give the compound a planar arrangement of 18 conjugated electrons, giving it a high electronic density and the presence of π bonds. Due to these characteristics, there is a strong absorption of phthalocyanine in the red region, which gives the intense blue color with the presence of a strong band in the region of 670 nm, called the Q band, with molar absorptivity (ε) on the order of 10^5 Lmol^{-1}cm^{-1} [105] and allows its application within the therapeutic window [106]. There are transitions of higher energy in the region of 350 nm, referring to the Soret band (band B), with a molar absorptivity (ε) of the order 10^4 Lmol^{-1}cm^{-1}. These intense bands occur due to transitions from the bonding orbital to the antibonding orbital ($\pi \rightarrow \pi^*$) [106,107]. The macrocyclic ring can strongly coordinate metallic centers, such as zinc, silicon, aluminum, and ruthenium, inside the macrocycle to give metallophthalocyanines (Figure 5) [102,108,109].

Metal ions such as ruthenium(II) or ruthenium(III) generally produce hexa-coordinate complexes, which allow for the binding of two ligands in axial position when they are coordinated to phthalocyanine [110]. It gives the opportunity to design compounds with appropriate conformational structures to drive subcellular localization as well as produce radical molecules by activation with light irradiation. With the aim of understanding the relationship between structure and activity, different ruthenium-phthalocyanine complexes were synthesized in our group (Figure 6), and their cytotoxicity was tested against different cancer cell lines. All the nitrosyl ruthenium-phthalocyanine complexes release NO in a way dependent on the wavelength light irradiation (Figure 7), suggesting two different photochemical pathways (Scheme 1).

(a)   (b)

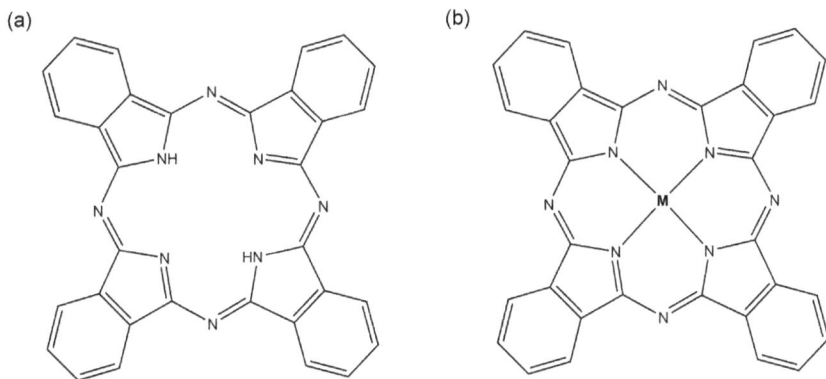

FIGURE 5 Chemical structure of phthalocyanines: (a) phthalocyanine free base and (b) metallophthalocyanine.

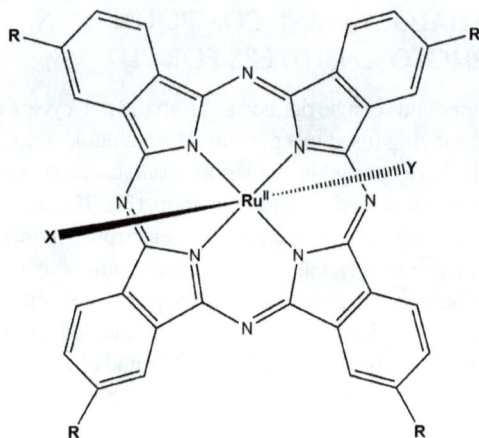

FIGURE 6   Molecular structure of *trans*-[RuX(Pc)Y] compounds.

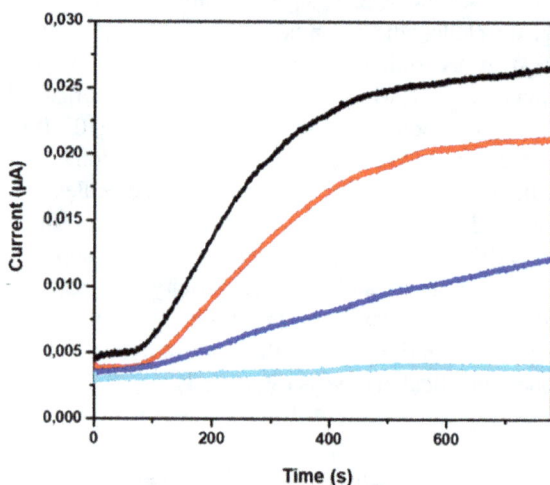

FIGURE 7   Chronoamperometric measurements for NO release of the *trans*-[RuNO (Pc-COO)NO$_2$] complex with light irradiation at (black) 377 nm; (red) 4,447 nm; (dark-blue) 532 nm; (light-blue) 660 nm.

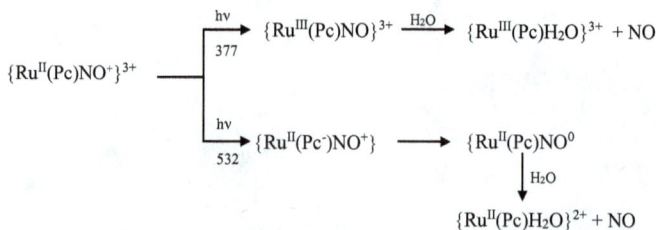

SCHEME 1   Photoreactivity of nitrosyl ruthenium-phthalocyanine complexes.

The cancer cell cytotoxicities of ruthenium-phthalocyanine complexes show interesting results and, so far, are highly intriguing. *In vitro* biological studies with ruthenium-phthalocyanine complexes demonstrate the high photocytotoxicity of these complexes, making them promising compounds as photosensitizing agents in PDT. Photon absorption for the subsequent formation of cytotoxic singlet oxygen ($^1O_2$) occurs through energy transfer between the triplet excited state of Ru-PS and oxygen present in cells. Due to their Q band, ruthenium-phthalocyanine compounds can initiate this process using radiation in the spectral region corresponding to 650 nm, which has the benefit of presenting low absorption of most biological chromophores. Photocytotoxicity by two ruthenium-phthalocyanine complexes such as *trans*-[Ru(NO)(Pc)(ONO)] and *trans*-[RuCl(Pc)(DMSO)] in the A-375 cancer cell line illustrates the effect of light irradiation in this class of compounds (Figure 8).

The highest cytotoxicity observed for the *trans*-[Ru(NO)(Pc)(ONO)] complex was attributed to a synergistic effect between NO and $^1O_2$. Figure 9 shows the

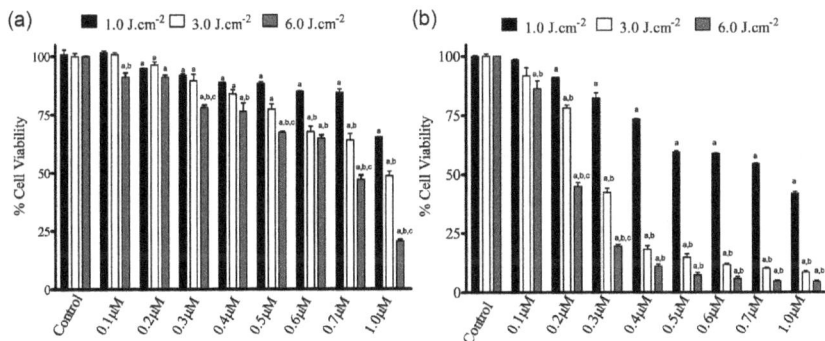

FIGURE 8 Photocytotoxicity of (a) *trans*-[RuCl(Pc)DMSO] and (b) *trans*-[RuNO(Pc) ONO] in the A375 cancer cell line under different irradiation light doses [111].

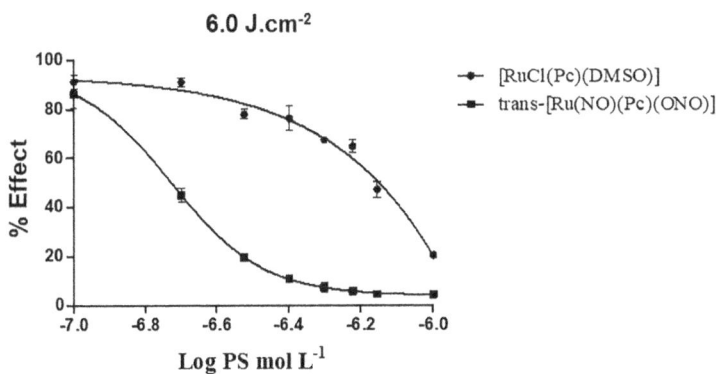

FIGURE 9 EC_{50} plot for *trans*-[Ru(NO)(Pc)(ONO)] (square) and *trans*-[RuCl(Pc) (DMSO)] (circle) complexes after light irradiation at 660 nm with a 6 J/cm^2 dose in the A375 cancer cell line. The cytotoxicity was measured after 4 hours of incubation [111].

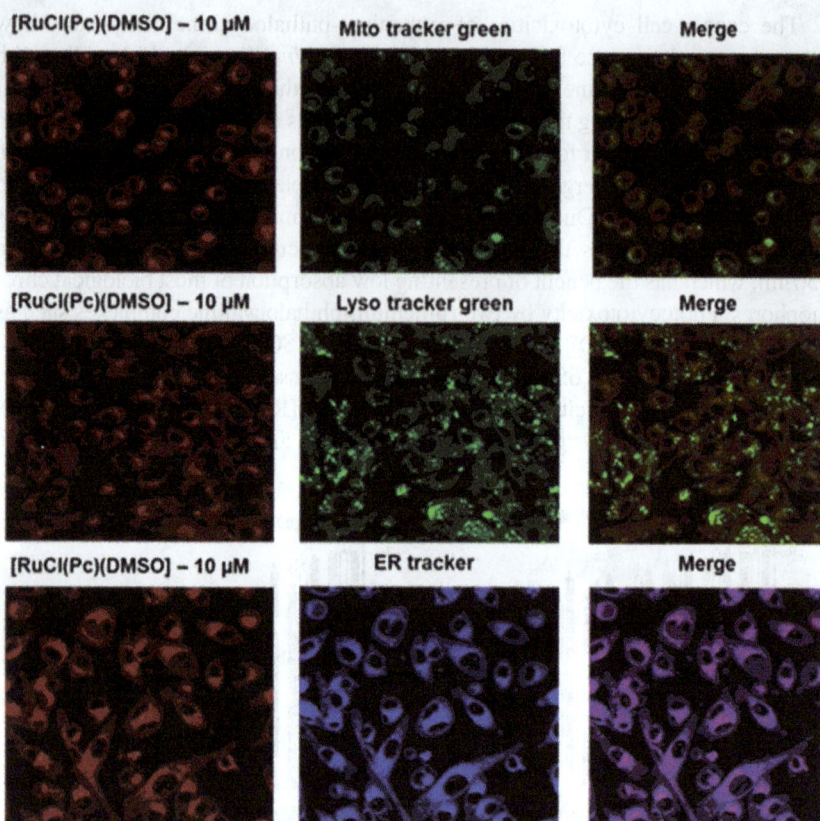

FIGURE 10 Confocal analysis of the ruthenium-phthalocyanine compound suggests subcellular localization on ER [111].

concentration-effect curve at 6.0 J/cm^2 light doses of both ruthenium-phthalocyanine complexes.

The confocal images (Figure 10) showed that indeed *trans*-[RuCl(Pc)(DMSO)] compound homed into the subcellular endoplasmic reticulum (ER) in A375 cancer cells over 4 hours. It is important to point out that ER has been proven to play a key role in some cancer development [112].

Measuring DNA modifications by comet assay (Figure 11), also called single-cell gel electrophoresis, could determine that a biological mechanism is involved in the cytotoxicity of the ruthenium complexes. The results seem to include direct action of the generated molecule radicals on DNA. In the presence of light irradiation, both complexes presented genotoxicity.

Despite these promising findings, further investigations are necessary to fully explore the potential of these complexes, including their mechanisms of action and possible applications. In addition to these examples, other ruthenium-phthalocyanine complexes have already demonstrated efficacy by releasing NO when subjected to light irradiation. An example of this type of complex is

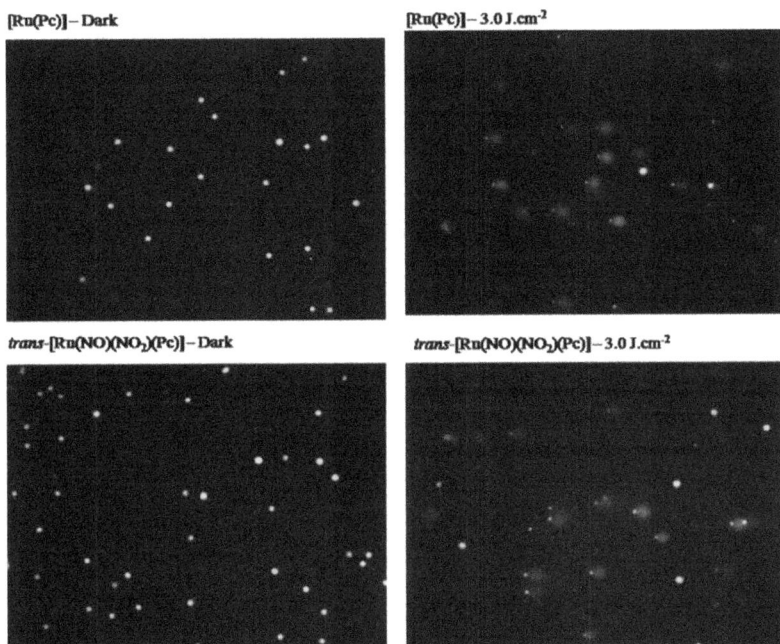

FIGURE 11   Comet assay of A375 cell line exposure to 0.5 μM of *trans*-[RuCl(Pc) (DMSO)] and *trans*-[RuNO(Pc)ONO] after 660 nm light irradiation [111].

$[Ru(pc)(pz)_2\{Ru(bpy)_2NO\}_2](PF_6)_6$, which stands out for its high production of $^1O_2$ (Tables 2 and 3). Cytotoxicity tests carried out with this compound, using the B16F10 melanoma cells, revealed that, at a concentration of 4 μM, when incubated for 4 hours and after irradiation at 660 nm with 5 J/cm² as a dose, it has the capacity to reduce cell viability to 21.0%, while the compound [RuPc] reduced to 80.0% under the same conditions used [113]. Another functional aspect of the use of ruthenium-phthalocyanine complexes is the possibility of using different axial ligands coordinated to Ru to improve photochemical properties and allow strategies to modulate cytotoxicity. The *in vitro* comparative study of the cytotoxicity between *trans*-[RuCl(Pc)DMSO] and *trans*-[Ru(Pc) (4-ampy)₂] (4-ampy = 4-aminopyridine) complexes against the murine melanoma cell line B16F10 demonstrated the great influence of the axial ligand. The complexes were incubated for 24 hours, and after that, the cells received an irradiation dose of 5.95 J/cm² at a wavelength of 660 nm. The results revealed that the *trans*-[RuCl(Pc)DMSO] complex reduced the viability to 9.32% ± 4.00% at the 0.5 μmol/L concentration and 6.43% ± 2.38% at the 1 μmol concentration/L. For the *trans*-[Ru(Pc)(4-ampy)₂] complex, the values were 51.37% ± 14.00% and 29.62% ± 8.09%, respectively [110]. Although all the ruthenium-phthalocyanine complexes are $^1O_2$ producing agents under light irradiation at 660 nm (Table 3), the relationship with cell viability is poor, and the cytotoxicity seems to be more related to cellular sublocalization.

TABLE 3
Quantum Yields of Singlet Oxygen Production for the
Ruthenium Complexes in Air Saturated DMSO

Complexes	Φ_Δ in the free form
trans-[RuCl(Pc)DMSO]	0.62
trans-[Ru(Pc)(4-ampy)$_2$]	0.14
[Ru(NO)(ONO)(pc)]	0.22
[Ru(pc)(pz)$_2${Ru(bpy)$_2$NO}$_2$]$^{6+}$	0.80
[Ru(Pc-DCBz)]	0.24
Na$_2$[RuCl$_2${pc-(COOH)}]	0.24
Na$_2$[RuCl$_2${pc-(COOH)$_4$}]	0.16
K$_6$[RuCl$_2${pc-(COO$^-$)$_4$}]	0.25
K$_4$[RuNOCl{pc-(COO$^-$)$_4$}]	0.16
[Rupc]	0.38

4 LIPOSOME AS A DRUG DELIVERY SYSTEM FOR THE RUTHENIUM-PHTHALOCYANINE COMPOUNDS

Among several drug delivery systems, liposomes present characteristics to be used in PDT due to their flexible physicochemical and biophysical properties, resulting in minimal adverse reactions. They are composed of a (phospho)lipid-based enclosing an interior aqueous space (Figure 12). It allows encapsulation within liposomes in either the aqueous compartment or within the lipid bilayer, depending on the solubility of the active compound. Some ruthenium-phthalocyanine derivative compounds have been liposome-entrapped, which improved the cancer cell cytotoxicity results.

The effect of the liposome can be better evidenced in the graphs in Figure 13. Clearly, the cytotoxicity of the compound used is not observed when dissolved in an aqueous solution. However, when encapsulated and subjected to light irradiation, it is possible to observe a substantial increase in cytotoxicity, probably due to an increase in cellular uptake. This shows the need to use a drug release system to increase the effectiveness of the compounds used. Most likely, in an aqueous solution, the carboxylate groups from phthalocyanine should be involved in hydrogen bond interactions with the cell membrane, which would prevent adequate cell sublocalization and consequently low cytotoxicity of the ruthenium compounds.

5 CONCLUSIONS AND FUTURE PERSPECTIVES

In this chapter, we have included fundamental bases for the use of ruthenium-phthalocyanine complexes as photosensitizers for cancer treatment. Despite the very significant results described for the coordination compounds based on ruthenium(II) species, there is still much to be done. Understanding the synergistic

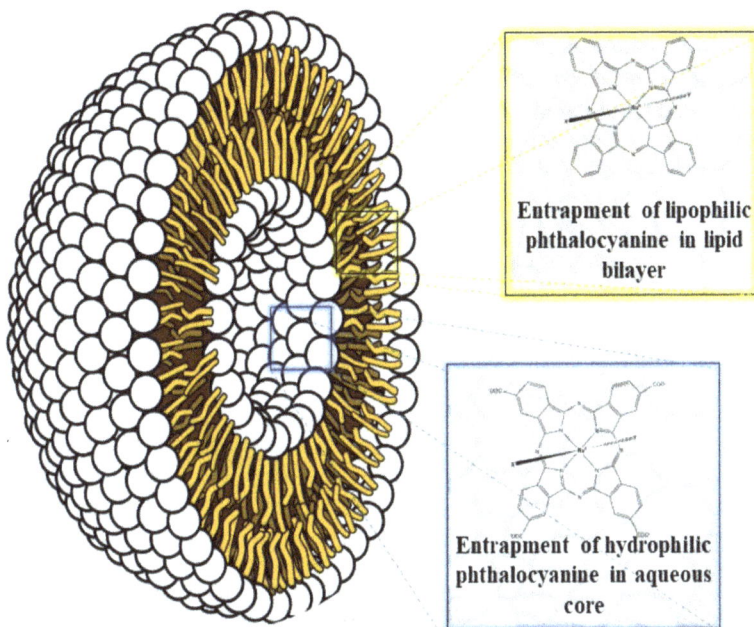

FIGURE 12 Liposome-entrapped phthalocyanine compounds as a model for drug delivery systems.

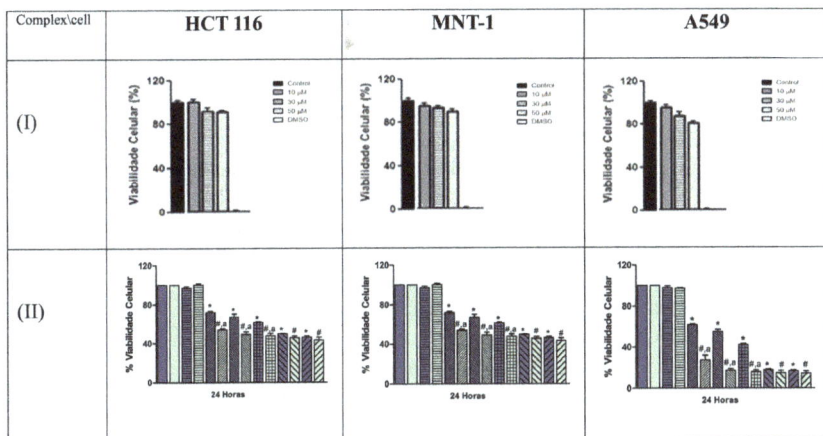

FIGURE 13 Cytotoxicity of a ruthenium-phthalocyanine complex, the *trans*-K_4[RuNO (PC-COO)Cl]: (a) aqueous solution in A549 cancer cell line in the presence of irradiation (660 nm; 2.97 J/cm^2), at different concentrations, and (b) liposome entrapped in A549 cancer cell line in the absence and in the presence of irradiation (660 nm; 2.97 J/cm^2), at different concentrations (8.10^{-5}; $1.6.10^{-4}$; $7.8.10^{-4}$; $1.57.10^{-3}$; $3.14.10^{-3}$ µM). Symbols used: * (different from dark control), # (different from light control), and a (different from respective dark control) (adapted from: [114]).

effect of NO and the rule related to the increase in the photocytotoxicity of ROS is a challenge to be overcome. *In vivo* assays should be an essential step to push the use of this kind of coordination compound forward from the design to clinical application. The ruthenium-phthalocyanine compounds promise to turn coordination compounds into a new generation of anticancer drugs.

ABBREVIATIONS AND DEFINITIONS

4-ampy	4-aminopyridine
DMSO	dimethylsulfoxide
ER	endoplasmic reticulum
PC	phthalocyanine
PDT	photodynamic therapy
PS	photosensitizer
ROS	reactive oxygen species

REFERENCES

1. J. Liu, H. Lai, Z. Xiong, B. Chen, T. Chen, *Chem. Commun.* **2019**, *55*, 9904–9914.
2. S. Monro, K. L. Colón, H. Yina, J .Roque III, P. Konda, S. Gujar, R. P. Thummel, L. Lilge, C. G. Cameron, S. A. McFarland, *Chem. Rev.* **2019**, *119*, 797–828.
3. P. Agostinis, K. Berg, K. A. Cengel, T. H. Foster, A. W. Girotti, S. O. Gollnick, S. M. Hahn, M. R. Hamblin, A. Juzeniene, D. Kessel, M. Korbelik, J. Moan, P. Mroz, D. Nowis, J. Piette, B. C. Wilson, J. Golab, *CA Cancer J. Clin.* **2012**, *61*, 250–281.
4. R. R. Allison, V. S. Bagnato, C. H. Sibata, *Future Oncol.* **2010**, *6*, 929–940.
5. R. R. Allison, K. Moghissi, *Clin. Endosc.* **2013**, *46*, 24–29.
6. E Cabuy, *Reliab. Cancer Ther. Energy-based Ther.* **2012**, *3*, 1–54.
7. A. P. Castano, T. N. Demidova, M. Hamblin, *Photodiagnosis Photodyn. Ther.* **2004**, *1*, 279–293.
8. B. C. Wilson, *Can. J. Gastroenterol.* **2002**, *16*, 393–396.
9. C. Imberti, P. Zhang, H. Huang, P. J. Sadler, *Angew. Chemie - Int Ed.* **2020**, *59*, 61–73.
10. R. L. Yanovsky, D. W. Bartenstein, G. S. Rogers, S. J. Isakoff, S. T. Chen, *Photodermatol Photoimmunol Photomed.* **2019**, *35*, 295–303.
11. H. Abrahamse, M. R. Hamblin, *Biochem. J.* **2017**, *473*, 347–364.
12. E. R. Da Silva, E. P. Dos Santos, E. Ricci-Júnior, *Rev. Bras. Farm.* **2009**, *90*, 211–217.
13. K. T. de Oliveira, J. M. de Souza, N. R. S. Gobo, F. F. de Assis, T. J. Brocksom, *Rev. Virtual. Quim.* **2015**, *7*, 310–335.
14. S. Monro, K. L. Colón, H. Yin, J. Roque, P. Konda, S. Gujar, R. P. Thummel, L. Lilge, C. G. Cameron, S. A. McFarland, *Chem. Rev.* **2019**, *119*, 797–828.
15. J. Deng, H. Li, M. Yang, F. Wu, *Photochem. Photobiol. Sci.* **2020**, *19*, 905–912.
16. S. Şener, A. Tahir Bayraç, B. Bilgenur Şener, C. Tozlu, N. Acar, B. Salih, M. Yüksel, Ö. Bekaroğlu, *Eur. J. Pharm. Sci.* **2019**, *129*, 124–131.
17. N. M. M. Moura, K. A. D. F. Castro, J. C. Biazzotto, J. A. Prandini, C. Lodeiro, M. A. F. Faustino, M. M. Q. Simões, R. S. da Silva, M. G. P. M. S. Neves, *Dye. Pigment.* **2022**, *205*, 110501.
18. B. Marydasan, R. R. Nair, P. S. Saneesh Babu, D. Ramaiah, S. Asha Nair, *ACS Omega.* **2019**, *4*, 12808–12816.

19. D. Lazewski, M. Kucinska, E. Potapskiy, J. Kuzminska, A. Tezyk, L. Popenda, S. Jurga, A. Teubert, Z. Gdaniec, J. Kujawski, K. Grzyb, T. Pedzinski, M. Murias, M. Wierzchowski, *Int. J. Mol. Sci.* **2022**, *23*, 10029.
20. W. Li, Q. Xie, L. Lai, Z. Mo, X. Peng, E. Leng, D. Zhang, H. Sun, Y. Li, W. Mei, S. Gao, *Photodiagnosis Photodyn. Ther.* **2017**, *18*, 83–94.
21. M. He, F. Du, W. Y. Zhang, Q.-Y. Yi, Y.-J. Wang, H. Yin, L. Bai, Y.-Y. Gu, Y.-J. Liu, *Polyhedron* **2019**, *165*, 97–110.
22. K. Plaetzer, B. Krammer, J. Berlanda, F Berr, T Kiesslich, *Lasers Med. Sci.* **2009**, *24*, 259–268.
23. V. Petrova, M. Annicchiarico-Petruzzelli, G. Melino, I. Amelio, *Oncogenesis* **2018**, *7*, 10.
24. S. Mallidi, S. Anbil, A. L. Bulin, G. Obaid, M. Ichikawa, T. Hasan, *Theranostics* **2016**, *6*, 2458–2487.
25. Lange C, Lehmann C, Mahler M, P. J. Bednarski, *Cancers* **2019**, *11*, E702.
26. F. Sajjad, N. Sun, T. Chen, Y.-J. Yan, D. Margetić, Z.-L. Chen, *Photodermatol. Photoimmunol. Photomed.* **2021**, *37*, 296–305.
27. E. Oakley, D. Bellnier, A. Hutson, H. Cooper, M. Habitzruther, S. Sexton, L. Curtin, L. Tworek, M. Mallory, B. Henderson, G. Shafirstein, *Photochem. Photobiol.* **2020**, *96*, 397–404.
28. Y. Mae, T. Kanda, T. Sugihara, T. Takata, H. Kinoshita, T. Sakaguchi, T. Hasegawa, R. Tarumoto, M. Edano, H. Kurumi, Y. Ikebuchi, K. Kawaguchi, H. Isomoto, *Mol. Clin. Oncol.* **2020**, *13*:1–6.
29. Y. Hanada, S. P. Pereira, B. Pogue, E. V. Maytin, T. Hasan, B. Linn, T. Mangels-Dick, K. K. Wang, *Gastrointest. Endosc.* **2021**, *94*, 179–186.
30. J. Kim, J. Kim, H. Yoon, Y.-J. Chae, K. Rhew, J.-E. Chang, *Curr. Issues Mol. Biol.* **2023**, *45*, 2474–2490.
31. I. O. de Albuquerque, J. Nunes, J. P. Figueiró Longo, L. A. Muehlmann, R. B. Azevedo, *Photodiagnosis Photodyn. Ther.* **2019**, *27*, 428–432.
32. J. Bartosińska, P. Szczepanik-Kułak, D. Raczkiewicz, M. Niewiedziol, A. Gerkowicz, D. Kowalczuk, M. Kwaśny, D. Krasowska, *Pharmaceutics* **2022**, *14*, 346.
33. K. Mahmoudi, K. L. Garvey, A. Bouras, G. Cramer, H. Stepp, J. G. Jesu Raj, D. Bozec, T. M. Busch, C. G. Hadjipanayis, *J. Neurooncol.* **2019**, *141*, 595–607.
34. L. Shi, P. Liu, J. Liu, Y. Yang, Q. Chen, Y. Zhang, H. Zhang, X. Wang, *Transl. Biophotonics.* **2020**, *2*, e201900028.
35. S. Hosokawa, G. Takahashi, K. Sugiyama, S. Takebayashi, J. Okamura, Y. Takizawa, H. Mineta, *Photodiagnosis Photodyn. Ther.* **2020**, *29*, 101627.
36. P. Vallecorsa, G. Di Venosa, G. Gola, D. Sáenz, L. Mamone, A. J. MacRobert, J. Ramírez 2, Adriana Casas, *J. Photochem. Photobiol. B Biol.* **2021**, *221*, 112244.
37. J. S. Souris, L. Leoni, H. J. Zhang, A. Pan, E. Tanios, H. M. Tsai, I. V. Balyasnikova, M. Bissonnette, C. T. Chen, *Nanomaterials* **2023**, *13*, 673.
38. Ł. Lamch, J. Kulbacka, M. Dubińska-Magiera, J. Saczko, K. A. Wilk, *Photodiagnosis Photodyn. Ther.* **2019**, *25*, 480–491.
39. D. G. Vital-Fujii, M. S. Baptista. *Brazilian J. Med. Biol. Res.* **2021**, *54*, 1–11.
40. L. F. Morgado, A. R. F. Trávolo, L. A. Muehlmann, P. S. Narcizo, R. B. Nunes, P. A. G. Pereira, K. R. Py-Daniel, C.-S. Jiang, J. Gu, R. B. Azevedo, J. P. F. Longo, *J. Photochem. Photobiol. B Biol.* **2017**, *173*, 266–270.
41. H. P. Monteiro, E. G. Rodrigues, A. K. C. Amorim Reis, L. S. Longo Jr, F. T. Ogata, A. I. S. Moretti, P. E. da Costa, A. C. S. Teodoro, M. S. Toledo, A. Stern, *Nitric Oxide – Biol. Chem.* **2019**, *89*, 1–13.

42. L. M. B. Cangussu, L. R. de Souza, M. G. de Souza, R. S. M. Junior, L. A. Muehlmann, P. N. de Souza, L. C. Farias, S. H. S. Santos, A. M. B. de Paula 1, A. L. S. Guimarães, *Lasers Med. Sci.* **2022**, *37*, 2509–2516.
43. J. Du, T. Shi, S. Long, P. Chen, W. Sun, J. Fan, X. Peng, *Coord. Chem. Rev.* **2021**, *427*, 213604.
44. G. M. Z. F. Damke, E Damke, P. de Souza Bonfim-Mendonça, B. A. Ratti, L. E. de Freitas Meirelles, V. R. S. da Silva, R. S. Gonçalves, G. B. César, S. de Oliveira Silva, W. Caetano, N. Hioka, R. P. Souza, M. E. L. Consolaro, *Life Sci.* **2020**, *255*, 117858.
45. Y. Zheng, J. Ye, Z. Li, H. Chen, Y. Gao, *Acta Pharm. Sin. B.* **2021**, *11*, 2197–2219.
46. B. Praena, M. Mascaraque, S. Andreu, R. Bello-Morales, E. Abarca-Lachen, V. Rapozzi, Y. Gilaberte, S. González, J. A. López-Guerrero, Á. Juarranz, *Pharmaceutics* **2022**, *14*, 2364.
47. M. Garcia-Diaz, Y. Y. Huang, M. R. Hamblin, *Methods.* **2016**, *109*, 158–166.
48. G. Brahmachari, A. Bhowmick, I. Karmakar, *J. Org. Chem.* **2021**, *86*, 9658–9669.
49. J. Sun, X. Cai, C. Wang, K. Du, W. Chen, F. Feng, S. Wang, *J. Am. Chem. Soc.* **2021**, *143*, 868–878.
50. M. Rajendran, *Photodiagnosis Photodyn. Ther.* **2016**, *13*, 175–187.
51. N. Miyoshi, T. Igarashi, P. Riesz, *Ultrason. Sonochem.* **2000**, *7*, 121–124.
52. H. Zhang, X. T. Tian, Y. Shang, Y.-H. Li, X.-B. Yin, *ACS Appl. Mater. Interfaces* **2018**, *10*, 28390–28398.
53. A. Kumar, A. Mondal, M. E. Douglass, D. J. Francis, M. R. Garren, L. M. E. Bright, S. Ghalei, J. Xie, E. J. Brisbois, H. Handa, *J. Colloid. Interface Sci.* **2023**, *640*, 144–161.
54. X. Li, J. Wang, R. Cui, D. Xu, L. Zhu, Z. Li, H. Chen, Y. Gao, L. Jia, *Dye. Pigment.* **2020**, *179*, 108395.
55. A. M. A. Abdelgawwad, A. Monari, I. Tuñón, A. Francés-Monerris, *J. Chem. Inf. Model.* **2022**, *62*, 3239–3252.
56. M. Wierzchowski, D. Łażewski, T. Tardowski, M. Grochocka, R. Czajkowski, S. Sobiak, L. Sobotta, *J. Photochem. Photobiol. B Biol.* **2020**, *202*, 111703.
57. J. C. M. Bremner, *Cancer Metastasis. Rev.* **1993**, *12*, 177–193.
58. D. Wang, L. Niu, Z. Y. Qiao, D.-B. Cheng, J. Wang, Y. Zhong, F. Bai, H. Wang, H. Fan, *ACS Nano.* **2018**, *12*, 3796–3803.
59. L. Larue, T. Moussounda Koumba, N. Le Breton, B. Vileno, P. Arnoux, V. Jouan-Hureaux, C. Boura, G. Audran, R. Bikanga, S. R. A. Marque, S. Acherar, C. Frochot, *ACS Appl. Bio. Mater.* **2021**, *4*, 1330–1339.
60. M. S. Soumya, D Gayathri Devi, K. M. Shafeekh, S. Das, A. Abraham, *Photodiagnosis Photodyn. Ther.* **2017**, *18*, 302–309.
61. M. R. Hamblin, H. Abrahamse, *Molecules* **2018**, *23*, 1–18.
62. D. L. Vega, P. Lodge, J. L. Vivero-Escoto, *Int. J. Mol. Sci.* **2016**, *17*, 56.
63. Z. Liu, M. Wu, M. Lan, W. Zhang, *Chem. Sci.* **2021**, *12*, 9500–9505.
64. D. Topkaya, S. Y. Ng, Y. Bretonnière, D. Lafont, L. Y. Chung, H. B. Lee, F. Dumoulin, *Photodiagnosis Photodyn. Ther.* **2016**, *16*, 12–14.
65. J. Benine-Warlet, A. Brenes-Alvarado, C. Steiner-Oliveira, *Photodiagnosis Photodyn. Ther.* **2022**, *37*, 102622.
66. S. Friães, E. Lima, R. E. Boto, D. Ferreira, J. R. Fernandes, L. F. V. Ferreira, A. M. Silva, L. V. Reis, *Appl. Sci.* **2019**, *9*, 5414.
67. S. M. M. Lopes, M. Pineiro, T. M. V. D. Pinho e Melo, *Molecules.* **2020**, *25*, 3450.
68. Y. Y. Huang, A. Wintner, P. C. Seed, T. Brauns, J. A. Gelfand, M. R. Hamblin, *Sci. Rep.* **2018**, *8*, 1–9.

69. S. R. El-Gogary, M. A. Waly, I. T. Ibrahim, O. Z. El-Sepelgy, *Monatshefte für Chemie* **2010**, *141*, 1253–1262.
70. R. Li, L. Yuan, W. Jia, M. Qin, Y. Wang, *Lasers Surg. Med.* **2021**, *53*, 400–410.
71. Y. H. Shih, C. C. Yu, K. C. Chang, Y.-H. Tseng, P.-J. Li, S.-M. Hsia, K.-C. Chiu, T.-M. Shieh, *Pharmaceuticals.* **2022**, *15*, 488.
72. K. Hayashi, M. Nakamura, H. Miki, S. Ozaki, M. Abe, T. Matsumoto, T. Kori, K. Ishimura, *Adv. Funct. Mater.* **2014**, *24*, 503–513.
73. X. Wen, X. Zhang, G. Szewczyk, A. El-Hussein, Y.-Y. Huang, T. Sarna, M. R. Hamblin, *Antimicrob. Agents. Chemother.* **2017**, *61*, 10–1128.
74. M. Shahpouri, M. A. Adili-Aghdam, H. Mahmudi, M. Jaymand, Z. Amoozgar, M. Akbari, M. R. Hamblin, R. Jahanban-Esfahlan, *J. Control. Release.* **2023**, *353*, 1002–1022.
75. P. Zago LH de, S. R. de Annunzio, K. T. de Oliveira, P. A. Barbugli, B. R. Valdes, M. Feres, C. R. Fontana, *J. Photochem. Photobiol. B Biol.* **2020**, *209*, 111903.
76. Q. Yu, W, X. Xu, Y. H. Yao, Z.-Q. Zhang, S. Sun, J. Li, *J. Porphyr. Phthalocyanines* **2015**, *19*, 1107–1113.
77. Y. Sun, D. Zhao, G. Wang, Y. Wang, L. Cao, J. Sun, Q. Jiang, Z. He, *Acta Pharm. Sin. B.* **2020**, *10*, 1382–1396.
78. K. Graham, E. Unger. *Int. J. Nanomedicine* **2018**, *13*, 6049–6058.
79. N. B. Pepper, W. Stummer, H. T. Eich, *Strahlentherapie Onkol.* **2022**, *198*, 507–526.
80. P. Wardman, *Clin. Oncol.* **2007**, *19*, 397–417.
81. J. C. M. Bremner, J. K. Bradley, G. E. Adams, M. A. Naylor, J. M. Sansom, I. J. Stratford, *Int. J. Radiat. Oncol.* **1994**, *29*, 329–332.
82. G. Graschew, M. Shopova, *Lasers. Med. Sci.* **1986**, *1*, 181–186.
83. J. L. Ignarro, *Nitric Oxide: Biology and Pathobiology*, 1st Ed., Academic Press, San Diego, CA, **2000**.
84. S. Korde Choudhari, M. Chaudhary, S. Bagde, A. R. Gadbail, V. Joshi, *World J. Surg. Oncol.* **2013**, *11*, 1.
85. G. Ren, X. Zheng, M. Bommarito, S. Metzger, Y. Walia, J. Letson, A. Schroering, A. Kalinoski, D. Weaver, C. Figy, K. Yeung, S. Furuta, *Sci. Rep.* **2019**, *9*, 1–21.
86. Burke AJ, F. J. Sullivan, F. J. Giles, S. A. Glynn, *Carcinogenesis* **2013**, *34*, 503–512.
87. D. Wink, *Carcinogenesis.* **1998**, *19*, 711–721.
88. K. M. Miranda, L. A. Ridnour, C. L. McGinity, D. Bhattacharyya, D. A. Wink, *Inorg. Chem.* **2021**, *60*, 15941–15947.
89. V. Somasundaram, D. Basudhar, G. Bharadwaj, J. H. No, L. A. Ridnour, R. Y. S. Cheng, M. Fujita, D. D. Thomas, S. K. Anderson, D. W. McVicar, D. A. Wink, *Antioxidants Redox. Signal.* **2019**, *30*, 1124–1143.
90. A. Kamm, P. Przychodzen, A. Kuban-jankowska, D. Jacewicz, A. M. Dabrowska, S. Nussberger, M. Wozniak, M. Gorska-Ponikowska, **2019.**, *93*, 102–114.
91. R. Keshet, A Erez, *DMM Dis. Model. Mech.* **2018**, *11*, 1–22.
92. L. A. Ridnour, D. D. Thomas, C. Switzer, W. Flores-Santana, J. S. Isenberg, S. Ambs, D. D. Roberts, D. A. Wink, *Nitric Oxide* **2008**, *19*, 73–76.
93. P. K. M. Kim, R. Zamora, P. Petrosko, T. R. Billiar, *Int. Immunopharmacol.* **2001**, *1*, 1421–1441.
94. S. Huerta, S. Chilka, B. Bonavida, *Int. J. Oncol.* **2008**, *33*, 909–927.
95. P. A. Vidi, M. J. Bissell, S. A. Lelièvre, *Methods Mol. Biol.* **2013.**, *945*, 193–219.
96. S. Furuta, G. Ren, J. H. Mao, M. J. Bissell, *Elife.* **2018**, *7*, e26148.
97. B. L. Ricca, G. Venugopalan, S. Furuta, K. Tanner, W. A. Orellana, C. D. Reber, D. G. Brownfield, M. J. Bissell, D. A. Fletcher, *Elife.* **2018**, *7*, e26161.
98. S. Huerta, *Future Sci. OA.* **2015**, *1*, FSO44.

99. P. C. Ford. *Nitric Oxide – Biol. Chem.* **2013**, *34*, 56–64.
100. P. C. Ford, I. M. Lorkovic, *Chem. Rev.* **2002**, *102*, 993–1017.
101. Z. N. da Rocha, R. G. de Lima, F. G. Doro, E. Tfouni, R. S. da Silva, *Inorg. Chem. Commun.* **2008**, *11*, 737–740.
102. Z. A. Carneiro, J. C. B. De Moraes, F. P. Rodrigues, R. G. de Lima, C. Curti, Z. N. da Rocha, M. Paulo, L. M. Bendhack, A. C. Tedesco, A. L. B. Formiga, R. S. da Silva, *J. Inorg. Biochem.* **2011**, *105*, 1035–1043.
103. P. C. Ford, K. M. Miranda, *Nitric Oxide - Biol. Chem.* **2020**, *103*, 31–46.
104. S. A. Cicillini, A. C. L. Prazias, A. C. Tedesco, O. A. Serra, R. S. da Silva, *Polyhedron.* **2009**, *28*, 2766–2770.
105. D. Wöhrle, *Adv. Mater.* **1993**, *5*, 942–943.
106. N. Kobayashi, M. Togashi, T. Osa, K. Ishii, S. Yamauchi, H. Hino, *J. Am. Chem. Soc.* **1996**, *118*, 1073–1085.
107. M. Grobosch, C. Schmidt, R. Kraus, M. Knupfer, *Org. Electron.* **2010**, *11*, 1483–1488.
108. M. Durmuş, J. Y. Chen, Z. X. Zhao, T. Nyokong, *Spectrochim. Acta Part A Mol. Biomol. Spectrosc.* **2008**, *70*, 42–49.
109. H. M. Almuzafar, H. M. Ahmed, N. N. AlDuhaisan, A. M. Elsharif, H. Aldossary, S. Rehman, S. Akhtar, F. Alam Khan, *J. Saudi. Chem. Soc.* **2022**, *26*, 101436.
110. T. J. Martins, L. B. Negri, L. Pernomian, K. do Carmo Freitas Faial, C. Xue, R. N. Akhimie, M. R. Hamblin, C. Turro, R. S. da Silva, *Front. Mol. Biosci.* **2021**, *7*, 1–12.
111. L. B. Negri. Fotobiomodulação e óxido nítrico como estratégias para potencializar a ação antitumoral da terapia fotodinâmica mediada por rutênio-ftalocianinas: Aspectos químicos, bioquímicos e fotobiológicos. [Ribeirão Preto]: Universidade de São Paulo, **2020**. Doctoral thesis.
112. D. Xu, Z. Liu, M.-X. Liang, Y.-J. Fei, W. Zhang, Y. Wu, J.-H. Tang, *Cell. Commun. Signal.* **2022**, *20*, 174.
113. T. A. Heinrich, A. C Tedesco, J. M. Fukuto, R. S. da Silva, *Dalton Trans.* **2014**, *43*, 4021–4025.
114. L. C. B. Ramos, Avaliação do efeito sinérgico de óxido nítrico e oxigênio singleto produzidos por complexo rutênio-ftalocianina em células tumorais: *estudos* fotoquímicos, fotofísicos e medida de atividade citotóxica in vitro. [Ribeirão Preto]: Universidade de São Paulo, **2016**. Doctoral thesis.

4 Metal Complexes as Probes and Inhibitors of Metabolic Enzymes

Madeline Denison
Department of Chemistry
Wayne State University
Detroit, Michigan 48202, USA
mdenison@wayne.edu

Claudia Turro
Department of Chemistry and Biochemistry
The Ohio State University
Columbus, Ohio 43210, USA
turro@chemistry.ohio-state.edu

Jeremy J. Kodanko
Department of Chemistry
Wayne State University
Detroit, Michigan 48202, USA
Barbara Ann Karmanos Cancer Institute
Detroit, Michigan 48201, USA
jkodanko@wayne.edu

CONTENTS

DOI: 10.1201/9781003361756-4

ABSTRACT

Cytochrome P450 (CYP) enzymes are a superfamily of heme-based proteins responsible for the metabolism of endogenous and exogenous molecules. Metabolism of
endogenous molecules includes biosynthesis of steroid hormones and production
of fatty acid metabolites. Cytochrome P450 enzymes also play a dominant role in
the metabolism of exogenous molecules, including xenobiotics and drugs. Atypical
expression of CYPs can cause abnormal levels of biomolecules to be produced
or degraded, which is associated with many human diseases, including cancer.
Moreover, metabolism of drugs by CYPs lowers drug bioavailability and efficacy.
The overexpression of CYPs in tumors makes CYPs important target enzymes
for cancer treatment. Importantly, due to CYPs general role in drug metabolism,
pharmacokinetic investigations are crucial for putting safe drugs on the market.
Studying CYP enzymes can reveal varying drug responses among ethnic groups
due to altered CYP activity and the potential for dangerous drug-drug interactions.
Metal-based compounds show many attractive properties, including selectivity for
cancer versus normal cells and photoactivatable ligand dissociation, which can
enhance biomolecule targeting and cytotoxicity. Photoactivated prodrugs have the
potential to target CYPs with high spatial and temporal precision at disease sites
while not disturbing CYPs involved in other tissues. Additionally, phosphorescent
metal complexes can be used to probe CYP activity and potentially monitor drug
metabolism. While metal-based complexes serve as nontraditional inhibitors and
probes, this chapter entails their successful inhibition and monitoring of CYP
enzymes and their powerful advantages versus organic-based agents.

KEYWORDS

Cytochrome P450; Drug Metabolism; Cancer; Photochemotherapy;
Phosphorescent

1   INTRODUCTION

1.1   CYTOCHROME P450: CHARACTERISTICS AND ROLE

Cytochrome P450 (CYP) is a superfamily of enzymes composed of 57 individual
human CYP genes, generally located in the liver and in some extrahepatic areas
[1–6]. Individual isoforms are classified by their family and subfamily [1–6]. For
example, CYP11A1 is isoform 1 of subfamily A of family 11 [7]. Among a family,
at least 59% of the sequence identity is shared, and among a subfamily, at least
70% is shared [7]. In contrast, percentages of shared sequence identity can be as
low as 16% between CYPs of different families [7].

CYPs are characterized by 12 helices with a heme in between helices I and L
[7]. When carbon monoxide binds to the heme, a strong absorption peak is present
at 450 nm, hence the name cytochrome "P450" [8]. The heme-iron cofactor acts as
a catalyst for CYP's main function: metabolism. When a substrate is held in close
proximity to the heme-iron cofactor by the enzyme, a series of redox reactions can
occur, resulting in oxidation of the substrate. Oxidation reactions include hydroxylation, epoxidation, and N- and O-dealkylation [9,10]. These reactions make exogenous molecules, like drugs, more polar and water-soluble, which can help drive

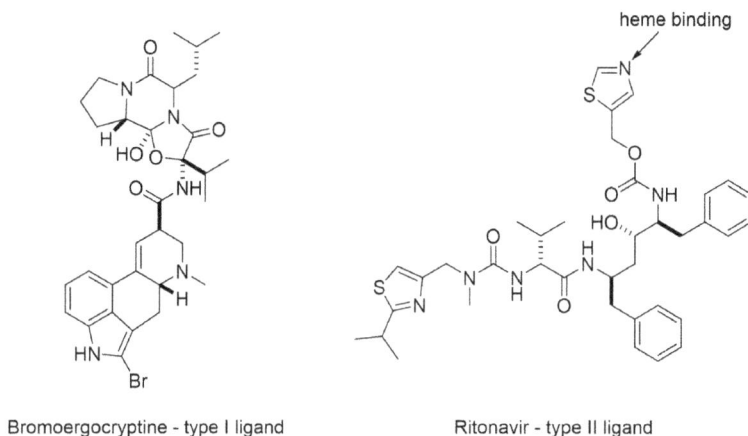

Bromoergocryptine - type I ligand   Ritonavir - type II ligand

FIGURE 1   Type I and II ligands of CYP.

their excretion from the body. CYPs also metabolize many endogenous molecules. For example, CYPs produce bile acid, steroid hormones, cholesterol, and thromboxane A2 and metabolize fatty acids, eicosanoids, and vitamins [3,5,11].

Although inhibitors of CYP enzymes vary widely in their size and structure, CYP inhibitors are generally divided into two categories: type I and type II ligands (Figure 1). Type I ligands inhibit CYPs by binding non-covalently within the active site and blocking access of substrates to the heme cofactor. Because type I ligands do not bind to the heme-iron center directly, these inhibitors can become oxidized. In contrast, type II ligands contain a nitrogen donor atom that binds tightly to the heme-iron center; because of this, type II inhibitors are generally resistant to oxidation [12]. Importantly, the type of inhibitor (I or II) can be determined easily by monitoring changes to the Soret band by electronic absorption spectroscopy. Ligand-free CYPs absorb at about 415 nm, and the displacement of iron-bound water leads to a spectral change depending on what kind of inhibitor or substrate is present [12]. Bromoergocryptine, a type I ligand, causes a blue shift in the maximum of the Soret band to 391 nm, whereas ritonavir, a type II ligand, causes a small red shift to 421 nm [12]. The sp^2 nitrogen feature of many type II ligands provides a useful handle for complexation with other metal centers, as described in this chapter.

1.2   INHIBITION OF CYPS AND CANCER

CYPs metabolize a wide range of endogenous molecules and are known to be overexpressed in various tumors [13–15]. While CYPs can promote oncogenesis through the formation of procarcinogens [16,17], overexpression of CYP enzymes can cause elevated levels of endogenous signaling molecules and lead to tumor progression. For example, CYP2J2 is responsible for converting arachidonic acid to epoxyeicosatrienoic acids, which drive angiogenesis and promote tumor growth [18,19]. Additionally, CYPs play an important role in producing steroids such as sex hormones; thus, CYP activity is also related to hormone-dependent cancers such as estrogen receptor-positive breast cancer [20–22] and prostate cancer [23].

CYP metabolism of exogenous and endogenous molecules plays an important role in cancer. Metabolites of endogenous molecules such as all-trans retinoic acid, a metabolite of vitamin A, and calcitriol, a metabolite of vitamin D, show protective effects against cancer [24, 25]. CYPs further oxidize these metabolites and deactivate them. Similarly, CYPs metabolize cancer drugs, leading to lower drug bioavailability and efficacy. For this reason, drug cocktails are commonly employed to reduce cancer drug metabolism. For instance, when docetaxel, an anticancer drug metabolized by CYP3A4, was evaluated in an orthotopic and immunocompetent mouse breast cancer model, a 30% shrinkage in tumor volume was observed. When docetaxel was used in combination with ritonavir (a potent and selective CYP3A4 inhibitor), a dramatic 70% decrease in tumor volume was achieved [26]. This evidence strongly supports CYP inhibition as an effective strategy to achieve better outcomes in cancer treatment.

Although CYP inhibition has been shown to increase the efficacy of some cancer therapies, CYP inhibition should be done selectively to avoid disruption of other vital CYP pathways. To achieve this goal, inhibitors that target CYPs specifically at tumor sites are needed. Common platinum-based anticancer drugs lack specificity for cancer cells, resulting in harmful side effects; however, recent metal-based complexes have emerged that show anticancer selectivity [27–30]. While these complexes are not designed to target CYP enzymes, it is important to note that they share anticancer properties; thus, metal scaffolds hold promise for further modification to inhibit CYPs expressed in tumors. Furthermore, metal-based compounds can be designed to release photolabile, biologically active ligands, including CYP inhibitors. This photorelease harnesses spatiotemporal control that could be used specifically at tumor sites. In this chapter, we will discuss research that has taken advantage of these characteristics to inhibit CYP enzymes for the treatment of cancer.

1.3   CYP PROBES

CYPs are best known for their role in drug metabolism. This vital pharmacokinetic event transforms drugs into more polar molecules to allow for clearance from the body. Importantly, while drugs are considered substrates of CYPs, drugs can also act as CYP inhibitors or inducers, which can lead to harmful drug-drug interactions. For example, amiodarone is an antiarrhythmic drug that inhibits CYP2C9. When taken in combination with warfarin, an anticoagulant metabolized by CYP2C9, warfarin levels are elevated, and risk of bleeding is increased [31]. The Food and Drug Administration (FDA) recommends drug-drug interaction studies to establish if investigational drugs act as inhibitors or inducers of a CYP enzyme and what CYP enzyme metabolites derived from new drugs are [32]. The FDA even suggests further study of metabolites of prospective drugs and their possible interaction with CYP enzymes [32]. Thus, tools for studying CYP activity are essential for providing the public with safe pharmaceuticals.

Another crucial feature that affects different CYPs is polymorphism. Single-nucleotide polymorphism is a mutation among CYP genes and can be shared among people from different ethnic backgrounds [3,4,11]. SNPs result in differences in the ability to metabolize drugs and can be detrimental to the efficacy of a drug. For example, 13%–23% of Asians are CYP2C19 poor metabolizers, leading to lower efficacy of drugs such as proton-pump inhibitors primarily metabolized by CYP2C19 [33]. In contrast, ultra-rapid metabolizers may metabolize a drug so quickly that it does not have a chance to elicit the desired effect. These differences in CYP metabolism abilities reinforce the importance of determining what CYP enzyme is responsible for the metabolism of individual drugs.

Methods to examine CYPs are vital for studying general CYP activity to determine the duration of metabolism, if one is a poor or ultra-rapid metabolizer, and to elucidate CYP induction and possible drug-drug interactions. Importantly, implementation of CYP probes in imaging experiments could indicate where metabolism is taking place. As previously mentioned, CYPs have been shown to be overexpressed in cancer and metabolize cancer drugs at tumor sites. Revealing the location of CYP metabolism can determine if a CYP inhibitor is needed to increase the localized concentration of a cancer drug or if another route of treatment is necessary.

Traditional studies of CYP activity involve high-performance liquid chromatography, which can measure the concentration of substrate and corresponding metabolites produced by CYP over time. A more convenient way of observing CYP activity involves exploiting the emissive properties of CYP substrates and probes [12]. Nonfluorescent substrates can be converted to fluorescent products by CYPs; thus, fluorescence is related to CYP activity. This is a common method to determine the inhibition of CYP activity and has also been used to image CYP activity in various cancer cell lines [34–36]. Although standard organic probes have been successful in analyzing CYP activity, metal-containing probes have emerged as advantageous tools due to their phosphorescent nature. While there are many examples of Ru(II) complexes being covalently attached to CYP enzymes to study mechanistic steps of metabolism [37–40], this chapter will focus on reversible and emissive metal-based CYP inhibitors that can be used as tools to probe CYP activity.

2   CYTOCHROME P450 INHIBITORS

2.1   Metal-Based Photocages

Photochemotherapy (PCT) involves the use of prodrugs known as photocages, which are biologically inert in the dark but release biologically active compounds upon irradiation (Scheme 1). Photocaging allows for control over when and where the drug is released. While organic photocleavable molecules have been developed, most organic-based photocaging groups are limited because they require UV light for photorelease, which cannot deeply penetrate tissue [41]. A more promising option is the use of metal complexes, which react with visible light. Since CYPs are known to metabolize both endogenous and exogenous molecules, it may not be desirable to inhibit both of these roles when treating cancer. Instead, spatiotemporal

Photochemotherapy (PCT)   **Small molecule activation**

photocaged compound   biological target

Photodynamic therapy (PDT)   **ROS generation**

photosensitizer   cell death

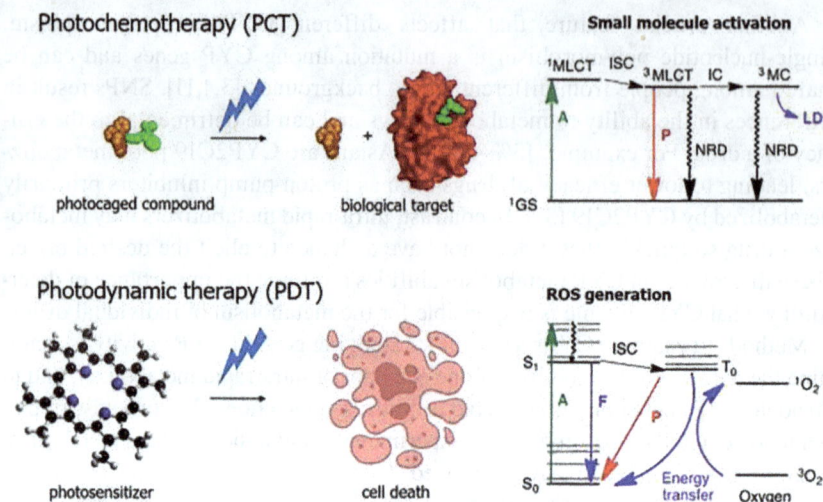

SCHEME 1   Photochemotherapy is described as a light-triggered activation of a prodrug to enable binding to its biological target. Irradiation of photocaged metal complexes for PCT allows for it to be excited to the singlet metal-to-ligand charge transfer state (^{1}MLCT), followed by intersystem crossing (ISC) to the triplet metal-to-ligand charge transfer (^{3}MLCT) and internal conversion (IC) to the triplet metal center (^{3}MC) finally resulting in ligand dissociation (LD). Specific energy levels of these states vary depending on the compound; energy levels are denoted arbitrarily as equal in this diagram. Photodynamic therapy (PDT) involves a photosensitizer that can produce singlet oxygen ($^1O_2$) or superoxide ($O_2^{\cdot-}$, not shown) to kill cancer cells. This is achieved by excitation to the singlet state, followed by ISC to the triplet state which can result in an energy transfer where $^1O_2$ is yielded from $^3O_2$. ^{1}GS = singlet ground state; A = absorbance; P = phosphorescence; NRD = nonradiative decay. Apoptotic cell graphic was created with BioRender.com.

control provided by photocages could allow for the release of CYP inhibitors, specifically in tumors. In the past decade, many ruthenium(II) complexes containing photocaged CYP inhibitors have been developed to take advantage of this idea.

The first example of a Ru(II)-based photocage containing a CYP inhibitor was in 2015 by Renfrew [42]. Ru(II) complexes were designed to contain econazole, a pan-CYP inhibitor that is used to treat cancer, mycobacterium tuberculosis, and leishmaniosis (Figure 2). Complex **1** containing two econazole ligands was found to be luminescent, whereas complex **2** with one ligand is non-luminescent, allowing for photosubstitution to be observed by confocal microscopy. Importantly, the toxicity of both complexes was tested in the dark and in the light on multiple cancer cell lines. Complex **1** was comparatively less toxic in the dark, while the light cytotoxicity of **1** and **2** was similar, giving **1** a more desired photoselectivity index (PI) as high as 34 in androgen-sensitive human prostate adenocarcinoma LNCaP cells.

Caged CYP11B1 inhibitors were designed by Glazer to contain etomidate and metyrapone (Figure 3) [43]. Metyrapone is used to treat Cushing's syndrome by inhibiting CYP11B1, also known as 11-beta-hydroxylase, thereby reducing cortisol in the adrenal glands [44]. Etomidate is used as a sedative; however,

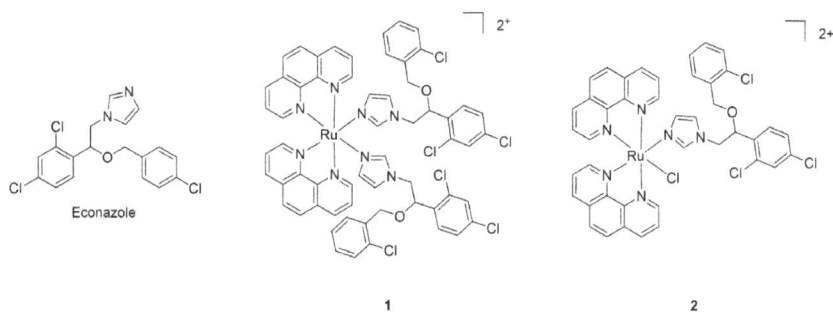

FIGURE 2   Pan-CYP inhibitor econazole and Ru(II) photocages containing 1 econazole ligand (**1**) and 2 econazole ligands (**2**) [42].

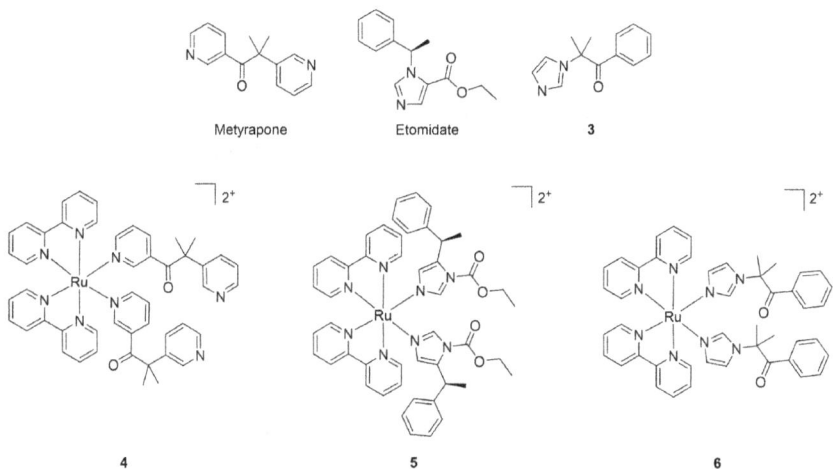

FIGURE 3   CYP11B1 inhibitors metyrapone, etomidate, and **3** complexed to Ru(II) photocages **4-6**.

it has been shown to reduce adrenal proliferation by inhibiting CYP11B1 [45]. A similar inhibitor **3** was also synthesized and complexed with the Ru(II) fragment Ru(bpy)$_2$ (bpy = 2,2'-bipyridine). Evidence of binding to CYP11B1 upon irradiation was confirmed by monitoring type II spectral shifts. Furthermore, the resultant Ru(II) complex was shown to produce DNA damage upon irradiation, as confirmed by inhibition of green fluorescent protein production. Glazer also synthesized Ru(II) complexes containing ligands based on the CYP1B1 inhibitor tetramethoxystilbene (Figure 4) [46]. CYP1B1 activates procarcinogens and metabolizes estradiol to 4-hydroxyestradiol, which is subsequently converted to estradiol 3,4-quinone, which can bind to DNA and act as a mutagen [47–49]. While Ru(II) complexes inhibited CYP1B1 in the micromolar range in the dark, irradiated Ru(II) complexes were much more potent, with **11** having a light IC$_{50}$ value of 310 pM and a PI value of 6,333. Because CYP1A1 is closely related in amino acid sequence to CYP1B1 and

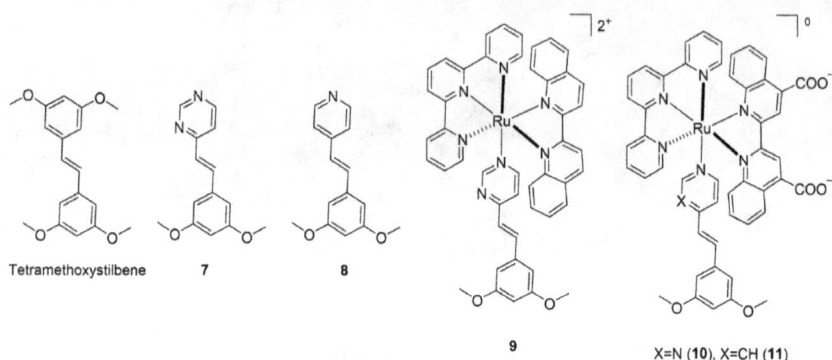

FIGURE 4 Ligands **7** and **8** modified from CYP1B1 inhibitor tetramethoxystilbene complexed to Ru(II) photocages **9-11** [46].

estradiol is a product of CYP19A1 while a substrate of CYP1B1, the selectivity of 1B1 was investigated. Lead compound **11** was found to be >100,000 times more selective for 1B1 over 1A1 and 62,800 times more selective for 1B1 over 19A1.

Kodanko and coworkers synthesized Ru(II) complexes containing abiraterone (ABI), a CYP17A1 inhibitor and agent approved by the FDA to treat castration-resistant prostate cancer (Figure 5) [50]. CYP17A1 is responsible for the steroidogenesis of dehydroepiandrosterone and androstenedione and is upregulated in prostate cancer [23]. Two Ru(II) photocaged analogs of abiraterone were prepared and evaluated for their ability to release ABI upon irradiation with visible light. The compound [Ru(tpy)(Me$_2$bpy)(ABI)]Cl$_2$ (**12**; tpy = 2,2′:2′,6″-terpyridine; Me$_2$bpy = 6,6′-dimethyl-2,2′-bipyridine) was shown to undergo photochemical release of ABI > four times more efficiently than **13**, [Ru(tpy)(biq)(ABI)]Cl$_2$ (biq = 2,2′-biquinoline) with λ_{irr} = 500 nm. When compound **12** was evaluated against CYP17A1, a K_d value of ~90 nM was obtained after irradiation with visible light, which is similar to the value observed for abiraterone, whereas no evidence of type II binding was observed under dark conditions. Importantly, **12** was also

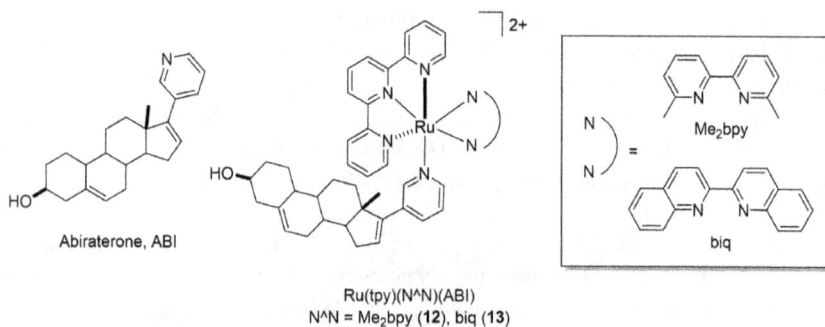

FIGURE 5 Ru(II) photocages containing CYP17 inhibitor abiraterone (ABI), where N^N = Me$_2$bpy (**12**) or N^N = biq (**13**) [50].

shown to induce photoactivated cell death in human prostate cancer DU145 cells, which express CYP17A1. Overall, the toxicity of **12** under light conditions in DU145 cells mirrored that of free ABI (EC$_{50}$ value of ~30 μM). Under dark conditions, the EC$_{50}$ value of **12** was >100 μM. This study proved that photocaging can be used to control the CYP binding and cytotoxic behavior of the FDA-approved prostate cancer drug ABI in cancer cells.

More recently, Kodanko and coworkers also synthesized and evaluated photocaged CYP3A4 inhibitors (Figure 6) and serendipitously discovered CYP3A4's affinity for metal-based fragments [51]. CYP3A4 is responsible for metabolizing the majority of pharmaceuticals and has been shown to be overexpressed in some cancers [6,26,52–54]. In this study, analogs **14–16** of the potent CYP3A4 inhibitor ritonavir were used as photolabile ligands that contain pyridyl groups known to bind in a type II fashion to the heme-iron center of CYP3A4 [55–57]. Photocaged analogs of compounds **14-16** were constructed using the fragments [Ru(tpy)(Me$_2$bpy], which is known for its PCT properties, and [Ru(tpy)(Me$_2$dppn]

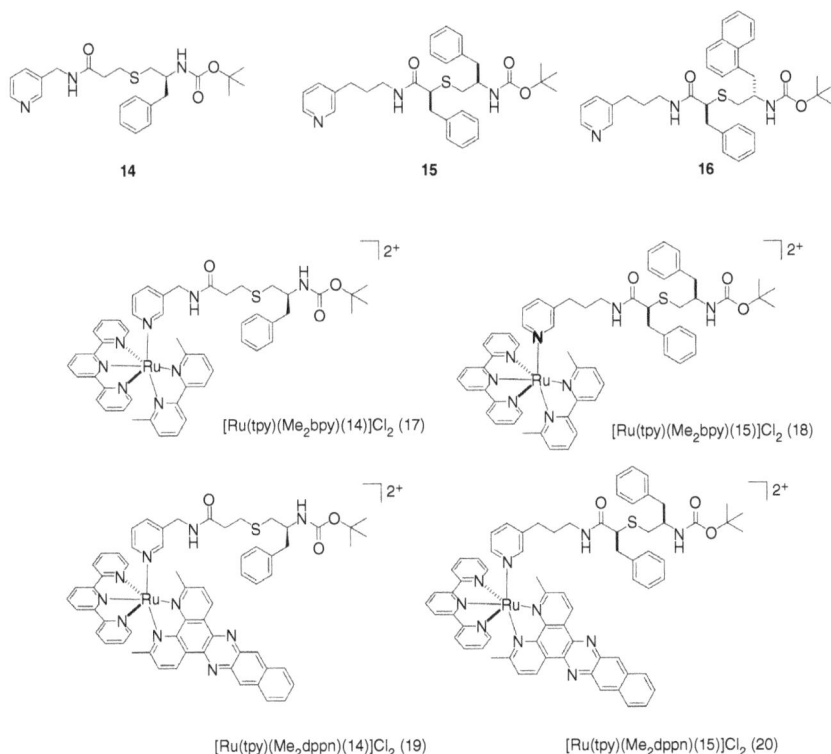

FIGURE 6 Ligands **14–16** based on CYP3A4 inhibitor ritonavir were complexed to various Ru(II) photocages varying in their bidentate ligands (Me$_2$bpy or Me$_2$dppn). Lead compound **17**, Ru(tpy)(Me$_2$dppn)(**14**) potently inhibited CYP3A4 in the dark and showed dual PCT/PDT properties [51].

(Me$_2$dppn = 3,6-dimethylbenzo[i]dipyrido[3,2-a:2′,3′-c]phenazine), which is known for its dual-action PCT and photodynamic therapy (PDT) behavior [58]. Similar to studies with CYP17A1 and the compounds described above, compounds **17** and **18** in this study derived from [Ru(tpy)(Me$_2$bpy)] were shown to undergo PCT behavior, namely photoactivated type II binding, upon irradiation with visible light. No evidence for type II binding was observed with compounds **17** and **18** under dark conditions. However, evaluation of compounds using CYP3A4 activity assays revealed that **17**, **19**, and **20** inhibit the enzyme more potently under dark conditions vs. light conditions, and more potently than the free inhibitors **14** and **15**. To confirm this surprising observation, compounds **17** and **18** were cocrystallized with CYP3A4, which revealed that the [Ru(tpy)(Me$_2$bpy)] fragments of **17** and **18** preferred to bind within a hydrophobic pocket in the substrate access channel. In these X-ray crystal structures, the pyridyl groups remain bound to Ru(II), while the organic inhibitors curl above the heme group. In an effort to establish the biological significance of these photocaged CYP3A4 inhibitors, an *in vitro* cell-based model system was examined, where synergy between a chemotherapeutic drug and an CYP3A4 inhibitor was observed in the past [59]. Importantly, lead compound **17**, a dual-action PCT/PDT compound, showed synergistic ability to kill DU145 cells when combined with the chemotherapeutic vinblastine, a drug that is metabolized by CYP3A4. Similar to the docetaxel-ritonavir drug cocktail, this synergy showed the importance of inhibiting CYPs to block cancer drug metabolism. It also showed for the first time that PCT, PDT, and a chemotherapeutic drug could be combined in a three-way cocktail to achieve synergistic effects.

Photoselective CYP inhibition and/or cytotoxicity is a powerful and potentially advantageous approach for controlling desired CYP inhibition. This targeted treatment by irradiation has the potential to eliminate side effects commonly associated with non-selective or toxic chemotherapeutic drugs. In particular, this approach has the potential to reduce the doses of chemotherapeutic drugs needed to achieve efficacy, which could reduce systemic side effects and drug resistance in cancer treatment. The ability to inhibit CYPs only in desired tissues, such as tumors, shows unique promise for treating cancer without disrupting CYPs participation in essential functions in other parts of the body, such as metabolism of various drugs or formation of endogenous molecules.

2.2 METAL-BASED CYP INHIBITORS

While the drug market is dominated by organic-based pharmaceuticals, metal-based therapeutics hold advantages that organic molecules do not. Scaffolds of organic drugs are limited by carbon, as tetrahedral carbon can only provide two stereoisomers, whereas octahedral metal centers can provide up to 30 stereoisomers [60–62]. Due to this unique geometry, metal complexes can be manipulated to mimic biologically active organic molecules while facilitating optimal spatial and electrostatic interactions within enzyme active sites [61,63,64]. Early metal-based therapeutics targeted DNA. Since then, researchers have taken advantage of the unique properties of metals to target various enzymes, such as kinases, proteases, glutathione S-transferase, acetylcholinesterase, and others [60,63,65]. Various metal-containing complexes have been developed to similarly target CYP enzymes.

Sanchez-Delgado and coworkers pioneered the design of metal-based compounds with anti-parasitic therapeutics for the treatment of Chagas disease caused by parasites like *Trypanosoma cruzi* and *Leishmania major* [66–70]. Metal precursors were complexed with azole derivatives such as ketoconazole and clotrimazole that are known as sterol biosynthesis inhibitors (Figure 7) that inhibit cytochrome P450$_{DM}$'s role in C14 demethylation of lanosterol to ergosterol (Scheme 2). Ergosterol is a main component that makes up the membranes of parasites; thus, inhibition of cytochrome P450$_{DM}$ results in decreased proliferation of *T. cruzi* and *L. major*. Lead Ru(II) compounds indeed showed an improvement in inhibition of parasite proliferation vs. the parent compound and were nontoxic in normal cells. Further investigation of the mechanism of action, however, demonstrated that Ru(II)-based complexes did not improve inhibition of sterol demethylation; rather, the enhanced cytotoxicity is most likely due to DNA intercalation.

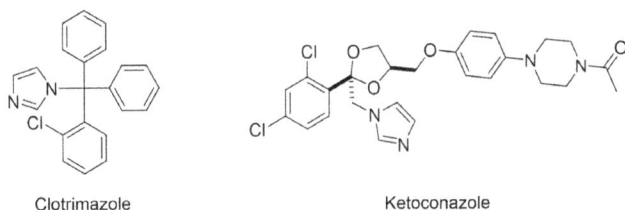

Clotrimazole   Ketoconazole

FIGURE 7   Sterol biosynthesis inhibitors (SBIs) that inhibit cytochrome P450$_{DM}$ included in various Ru(II) complexes to treat *Trypanosoma cruzi* and *Leishmania major* [66–70].

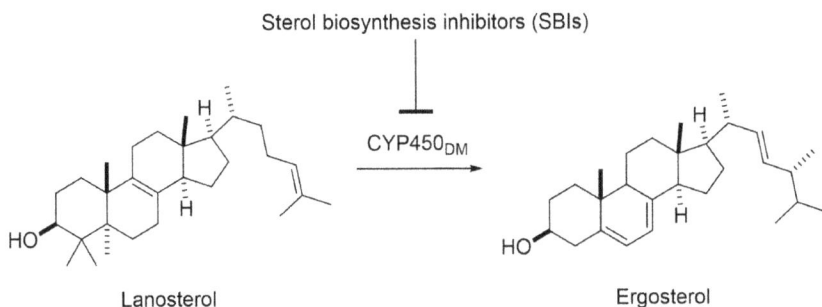

Sterol biosynthesis inhibitors (SBIs)

CYP450$_{DM}$

Lanosterol   Ergosterol

SCHEME 2   Lansosterol conversion by CYP450$_{DM}$ to ergosterol, the principal component of parasites membrane. This reaction can be inhibited by SBIs as seen in Figure 7.

CYP19A1, commonly named aromatase, is primarily responsible for catalyzing the conversion of testosterone to estradiol. Elevated levels of estradiol are related to estrogen receptor-positive breast cancer; as such, aromatase inhibitors (AIs) are generally given to postmenopausal women who no longer produce estrogen to inhibit estradiol production. Common AIs include exemestane, letrozole, and anastrozole (Figure 8). Coordination of AIs with transition metals began with the synthesis of letrozole, which formed a polymer to bind to copper(I) in a tetradentate fashion [71]. Metal-based letrozole complexes were expanded by Tang et al. to include copper(II), nickel(II), and cobalt(II), each with four monodentate letrozole ligands [71,72]. Castongua and coworkers have designed various organoruthenium(II) complexes containing letrozole or anastrozole [73–75]. While Ru(II) complexes did not show improved inhibition of aromatase activity from their corresponding AI drug, Ru(II) was more cytotoxic. Unfortunately, Ru(II) complexes showed no selectivity for tumor cells over normal cells. However, *in vivo* studies in zebrafish showed no significant mortality 96 hours after fertilization.

Another metal-based CYP19A1 inhibitor implemented a prodrug strategy where *trans*-$[PtCl(NH_3)_2(H_2O)]^+$ was conjugated to vitamin B12 (Figure 9) [76]. Platinum(II) coordinates to the nitrogen of the β-axial group of vitamin B12, and anastrozole or a known drug is added to displace chloride. In the cellular environment, the cobalt(III) center of B12 is reduced to cobalt(II), allowing for the release of the platinum drug-containing complex. While the anastrozole-containing complex was not extensively studied, a derivative containing cytarabine (for the treatment of myeloid leukemia and non-Hodgkin's lymphoma) showed release upon reduction with Zn^0.

Since the advent of cisplatin, many researchers have explored metal-based cancer therapeutics to overcome cisplatin resistance and improve cytotoxic selectivity in cancer cells. However, only a few have designed metal-based therapeutics that target CYP enzymes. While inhibition of certain CYPs by larger metal complexes may be unlikely due to varying active site cavities among CYPs, these complexes provide a promising approach to simultaneously inhibiting CYPs involved in human health, including infectious diseases and cancer, and eliciting cytotoxic effects through interactions with other biomolecules such as DNA.

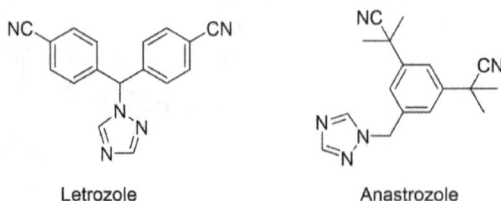

Letrozole   Anastrozole

FIGURE 8 Aromatase (or CYP19A1) inhibitors (AIS) complexed to Cu(II), Co(II), Ni(II), and Ru(II) to treat ER+ breast cancer [71–75].

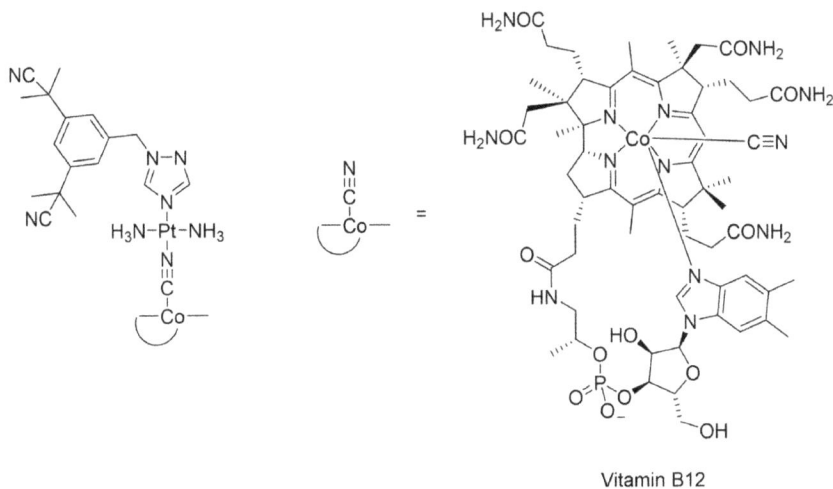

Vitamin B12

FIGURE 9 AI inhibitor anastrozole complexed to Pt(II) coordinated to the nitrogen of the β-axial group of vitamin B12 [76].

3   CYTOCHROME P450 PROBES

As mentioned above, a powerful property of metal-based complexes is phosphorescence. This phosphorescence results in remarkably longer-lived emission lifetimes, into the microsecond range, vs. nanoseconds for most fluorescent organic molecules. The long lifetimes of some transition metal compounds allow for the use of lifetime gating used in time-resolved emission spectroscopy or phosphorescent lifetime imaging microscopy, where emission can be gathered after a time point where background autofluorescence from endogenous biomolecules has decayed but phosphorescence persists. Metal-based probes have taken advantage of lifetime gating to increase signal-to-background ratios and accurately depict emission caused by probes. A few select examples include sensing of amino acids by Ir(III) [77,78], detecting oligonucleotides sequences by Ru(II) [79] and Ir(III) [80], and identifying solvent vapors by Re(I) [81]. Fortunately, this list of metal-based probes has expanded recently to include monitoring important CYP enzymes.

Gray and coworkers designed inhibitors of *Pseudomonas* putida P450$_{cam}$ (P450$_{cam}$), a prokaryotic CYP commonly used to study the oxidation mechanism of CYPs due to its similar sequence homology to eukaryotic CYPs [82–85]. Inhibitors included adamantane, ethylbenzene, and imidazole linked to Ru(II) complexes or dansyl fluorophores through an alkyl chain (Figure 10). Inhibitors displayed emission quenching when bound to the enzyme due to Förster energy transfer with the CYP active site heme (Scheme 3) [86–89]. Shorter distances between the Ru(II) center and the heme resulted in shorter excited lifetimes [87]. Also, docking and X-ray crystallographic studies demonstrated conformational changes where the substrate access channel opens to fit the inhibitor and the alkyl tether spans the active site with the Ru(II) center siting at the protein surface. While this work

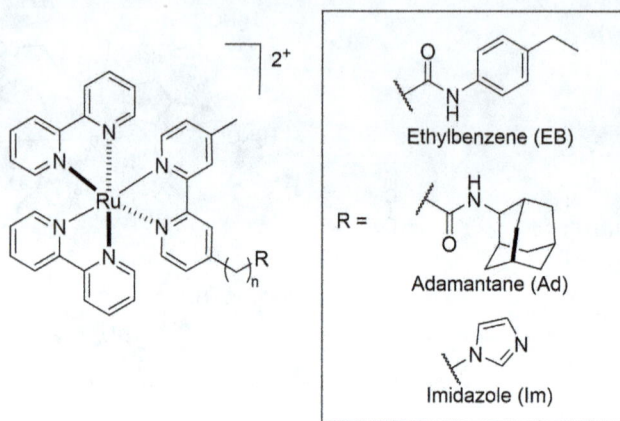

FIGURE 10   Ru(bpy)$_2$-based P450$_{cam}$ inhibitors [86–89].

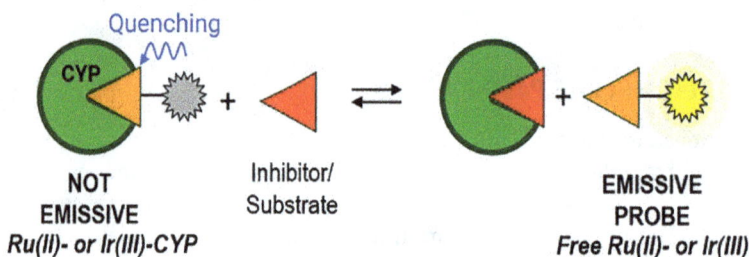

SCHEME 3   Emissive Ru(II) or Ir(III) complexes are quenched in CYP active site, however when a CYP inhibitor or substrate is added, Ru(II) or Ir(III) is displaced and emission is increased.

demonstrated the remarkable flexibility and conformational change of P450$_{cam}$ to accommodate an access channel for the large inhibitor, it also showed promise of emissive metal compounds to be used as active site probes [87, 88].

Kodanko and coworkers implemented a similar strategy with brightly emissive Ir(III)-based complexes that act as inhibitors and probes of the major drug-metabolizing enzyme CYP3A4. Initial studies demonstrated Ir(III)-based complexes with larger, hydrophobic ligands were more potent CYP3A4 inhibitors than Ru(II)-based analogs [90]. Thus, studies were continued designing a library of ten Ir(III)-based inhibitors with varying cyclometallating ligands (2-phenylquinoline (pq) 2-(2,4-difluorophenyl)pyridine (dfpp), and 2-(benzo[b]thiophen-2-yl)quinoline (btq), (Figure 11), seven of which were cocrystallized within the CYP3A4 active site [91]. The remaining bipyridyl ligand contained a six-atom tether with a terminal pyridine to anchor the complex to the heme. This ligand varied in

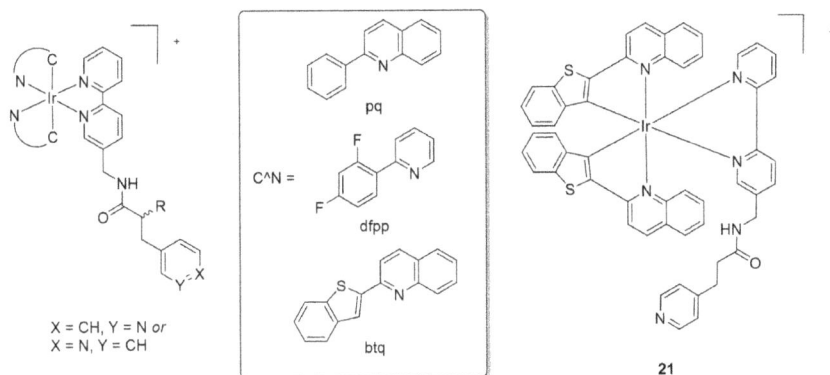

FIGURE 11   Ir(III)-based CYP3A4 inhibitor and lead compound Ir(btq)$_2$(L) **21** [91].

placement of the nitrogen of the terminal pyridine and implementation of hydrophobic side chains and corresponding stereochemistry on the side chains (L vs. D) and also at the metal center (Δ vs. Λ). Biological studies revealed complexes had low cellular toxicity, were selective for CYP3A4, and potent with K_d values as low as 9 nM. Importantly, complexes were brightly emissive and had long emission lifetimes. These initially emissive complexes become quenched in the CYP3A4 active site. Subsequent addition of a CYP3A4 inhibitor or substrate results in displacement of Ir(III) and an observed increase in emission. When the order of addition was reversed, emission decreased. Thus, CYP3A4 active site occupancy can be monitored dynamically by reversible changes in emission as confirmed by steady-state emission spectra and changes in the signature Soret band at 420 nm. Importantly, due to long-lived emission lifetimes, lifetime gating was used to show a signal-to-background ratio of 6 with 100 nM of lead compound **21**. Implementation of lifetime gating and consequent lower detection limits signifies lower concentrations of probe are necessary to obtain desired results, thereby reducing the risk of interference for nonspecific binding and cellular toxicity in future cellular assays.

Metal-based complexes have proven to be powerful tools in studying many different systems by taking advantage of their emissive characteristics and long-lived phosphorescent lifetimes, which allows for lifetime gating. The use of lifetime gating decreases detection limits by reducing background fluorescence and probe needed to monitor activity. Minimal probe concentration is optimal to reduce non-specific binding and toxicity so that probes can be developed for cellular and *in vivo* studies to monitor drug metabolism in real time. Thus, metal-based CYP probes are promising candidates for monitoring drug metabolism by means of a simple emission assay. Additionally, there are several reports of these probes used in live cell imaging, including the detection of hypoxia [92–95], hypochlorite [96], cysteine [97,98], and peroxynitrite [99]; therefore, it is possible metal-based probes have the potential to image CYP activity to determine where metabolism is taking place.

4   GENERAL CONCLUSIONS

CYPs are crucial enzymes in biology due to their role in biosynthesis, drug metabolism, and human disease states such as cancer. Metal-based inhibitors, especially those containing photocages, offer the promise to selectively inhibit CYPs within desired tissues. This selectivity has great potential to ensure CYPs outside of disease tissues such as the tumor microenvironment are not disturbed. Moreover, metal-based tools to monitor the active site occupancy of CYPs have emerged that exploit long-lived phosphorescent lifetimes to achieve lower detection limits in emission assays. The reversible quenching of emissive metal-based complexes provides access to simple emission assays that could conveniently monitor drug metabolism, drug-drug interactions, induction and CYP polymorphism dynamically over time. Reported successful photocaging, inhibition, and probing of CYP enzymes demonstrate the superior advantages of metal-based complexes over traditional inhibitors or probes and provides a bright future for metal-based complexes as novel therapeutics and chemical tools for monitoring CYPs.

ABBREVIATIONS AND DEFINTIONS

A	absorbance
ABI	abiraterone
AIs	aromatase inhibitors
biq	2,2'-biquinoline
bpy	2,2'-bipyridine
btq	2-(benzo[b]thiophen-2-yl)quinoline
CYP	cytochrome P450
dfpp	2-(2,4-difluorophenyl)pyridine
FDA	Food and Drug Administration
^{1}GS	singlet ground state
IC	internal conversion
^{3}MC	triplet metal center
Me$_2$bpy	6,6'-dimethyl-2,2'-bipyridine
Me$_2$dppn	3,6-dimethylbenzo[i]dipyrido[3,2-a:2',3'-c]phenazine
^{1}MLCT	singlet metal-to-ligand charge transfer state
^{3}MLCT	triplet metal-to-ligand charge transfer state
NRD	nonradiative decay
$^1O_2$	singlet oxygen
$O_2{}^{\cdot-}$	superoxide
$^3O_2$	triplet oxygen
P	phosphorescence
PCT	photochemotherapy
PDT	photodynamic therapy
P450$_{cam}$	*Pseudomonas* putida P450$_{cam}$
pq	2-phenylquinoline
tpy	2,2':2',6''-terpyridine

REFERENCES

1. S. N. de Wildt, G.L. Kearns, J. S. Leeder, J. N. van den Anker, *Clin. Pharmacokinet.* **1999**, *37*, 485–505.
2. J. H. Lin, A. Y. H. Lu, *Clin. Pharmacokinet.* **1998**, *35*, 361–390.
3. T. Lynch, A. Price, *Am. Fam. Physician* **2007**, *76*, 391–396.
4. U. M. Zanger, M. Schwab, *Pharmacol. Ther.* **2013**, *138*, 103–141.
5. M. Seliskar, D. Rozman, Biochim. Biophys. *Acta, Gen. Subj.* **2007**, *1770*, 458–466.
6. O. Lolodi, Y.-M. Wang, W. C. Wright, T. Chen, *Curr. Drug Metab.* **2018**, *18*, 1095–1105.
7. B. Meunier, S. P. de Visser, S. Shaik, *Chem. Rev.* **2004**, *104*, 3947–3980.
8. T. Omura, R. Sato, *J. Biol. Chem.* **1964**, *239*, 2370–2378.
9. E. M. Isin, F. P. Guengerich, *Biochim. Biophys. Acta, Gen. Subj.* **2007**, *1770*, 314–329.
10. A. P. Li, D. L. Kaminski, A. Rasmussen, *Toxicology* **1995**, *104*, 1–8.
11. A. M. McDonnell, C. H. Dang, J. *Adv. Pract. Oncol.* **2013**, *4*, 263–268.
12. I. F. Sevrioukova, T. L. Poulos, *Adv. Exp. Med. Biol.* **2015**, *851*, 83–105.
13. C. Rodriguez-Antona, M. Ingelman-Sundberg, *Oncogene* **2006**, *25*, 1679–1691.
14. R. D. Bruno, V. C. O. Njar, *Bioorg. Med. Chem.* **2007**, *15*, 5047–5060.
15. M. C. E. McFadyen, W. T. Melvin, G. I. Murray, Mol. Cancer Ther. **2004**, *3*, 363–371.
16. S. Sansen, J. K. Yano, R. L. Reynald, G. A. Schoch, K. J. Griffin, C. D. Stout, E. F. Johnson, *J. Biol. Chem.* **2007**, *282*, 14348–14355.
17. J. Sridhar, N. Goyal, J. Liu, M. Foroozesh, *Molecules* **2017**, 22, 1143
18. J. -G. Jiang, Y. -G. Ning, C. Chen, D. Ma, Z. -J. Liu, S. Yang, J. Zhou, X. Xiao, X. A. Zhang, M. L. Edin, J W. Card, J. Wang, D. C. Zeldin, D. W. Wang, *Cancer Res.* **2007**, *67*, 6665–6674.
19. A. A. Rand, A. Rajamani, S. D. Kodani, T. R. Harris, L. Schlatt, B. Barnych, A. G. Passerini, B. D. Hammock, *J. Lipid Res.* **2019**, *60*, 1996–2005.
20. H. J. Chan, K. Petrossian, S. Chen, *J. Steroid Biochem. Mol. Biol.* **2016**, *161*, 73–83.
21. S. Chumsri, T. Howes, T. Bao, G. Sabnis, A. Brodie, *J. Steroid Biochem. Mol. Biol.* **2011**, *125*, 13–22.
22. S. Daldorff, R. M. R. Mathiesen, O. E. Yri, H. P. Ødegård J. Geisler, *Br. J. Cancer* **2017**, *116*, 10–20.
23. A. B. Alex, S. K. Pal, N. Agarwal, Ther. Adv. *Med. Oncol.* **2016**, *8*, 267–275.
24. N. Siddikuzzaman, C. Guruvayoorappan, V. M. Berlin Grace, *Immunopharmacol. Immunotoxicol.* **2011**, *33*, 241–249.
25. L. Díaz, M. Díaz-Muñoz, A. García-Gaytán, I. Méndez, *Nutrients* **2015**, *7*, 5020–5050.
26. M. van Eijk, R. J. Boosman, A. H. Schinkel, A. D. R. Huitema, J. H. Beijnen, *Cancer Chemother. Pharmacol.* **2019**, *84*, 487–499.
27. S. Gupta, J. M. Vandevord, L. M. Loftus, N. Toupin, M. H. Al-Afyouni, T. N. Rohrabaugh, C. Turro, J. J. Kodanko, *Inorg. Chem.* **2021**, *60*, 18964–18974.
28. R. Pettinari, F. Marchetti, F. Condello, C. Pettinari, G. Lupidi, R. Scopelliti, S. Mukhopadhyay, T. Riedel, P. J. Dyson, *Organometallics* **2014**, *33*, 3709–3715.
29. G. H. Ribeiro, A. P. M. Guedes, T. D. de Oliveira, C. R. S. T. b. de Correia, L. Colina-Vegas, M. A. Lima, J. A. Nóbrega, M. R. Cominetti, F. V. Rocha, A. G. Ferreira, E. E. Castellano, F. R. Teixeira, A. A. Batista, *Inorg. Chem.* **2020**, *59*, 15004–15018.
30. K. M. Oliveira, E. J. Peterson, M. C. Carroccia, M. R. Cominetti, V. M. Deflon, N. P. Farrell, A. A. Batista, R. S. Correa, *Dalton Trans.* **2020**, *49*, 16193–16203.
31. L. D. Heimark, L. Wienkers, K. Kunze, M. Gibaldi, A. C. Eddy, W. F. Trager, R. A. O'Reilly, D. A. Goulart, *Clin. Pharmacol. Ther.* **1992**, *51*, 398–407.

32. U.S. Food and Drug Administration. In Vitro Drug Interaction Studies - Cytochrome P450 Enzyme- and Transporter-Mediated Drug Interactions Guidance for Industry (Accessed Feb 1, 2023 at https://www.fda.gov/regulatory-information/search-fda-guidance-documents/in-vitro-drug-interaction-studies-cytochrome-p450-enzyme-and-transporter-mediated-drug-interactions).
33. E. Chong, M. H. H. Ensom, *Pharmacotherapy* **2003**, *23*, 460–471.
34. J. Ning, T. Liu, P. Dong, W. Wang, G. Ge, B. Wang, Z. Yu, L. Shi, X. Tian, X. Huo, L. Feng, C. Wang, C. Sun, J. Cui, T. D. James, X. Ma, *J. Am. Chem. Soc.* **2019**, *141*, 1126–1134.
35. Z. -R. Dai, G. -B. Ge, L. Feng, J. Ning, L. -H. Hu, Q. Jin, D. -D. Wang, X. Lv, T. -Y. Dou, J. -N. Cui, L. Yang, *J. Am. Chem. Soc.* **2015**, *137*, 14488–14495.
36. J. Ning, Z. Tian, B. Wang, G. Ge, Y. An, J. Hou, C. Wang, X. Zhao, Y. Li, X. Tian, Z. Yu, X. Huo, C. Sun, L. Feng, J. Cui, X. Ma, *Mater. Chem. Front.* **2018**, 2, 2013–2020.
37. M. E. Ener, Y. -T. Lee, J. R. Winkler, H. B. Gray, L. Cheruzel, *Proc. Natl. Acad. Sci. U.S.A.* **2010**, *107*, 18783–18786.
38. J. Spradlin, D. Lee, S. Mahadevan, M. Mahomed, L. Tang, Q. Lam, A. Colbert, O. S. Shafaat, D. Goodin, M. Kloos, M. Kato, L. E. Cheruzel, *Biochim. Biophys. Acta, Proteins Proteomics* **2016**, *1864*, 1732–1738.
39. Q. Lam, M. Kato, L. Cheruzel, *Biochim. Biophys. Acta, Bioenerg.* **2016**, **1857**, 589–597.
40. N. -H. Tran, N. Huynh, T. Bui, Y. Nguyen, P. Huynh, M. E. Cooper, L. Cheruzel, *Chem. Commun.* **2011**, *47*, 11936–11938
41. P. Dunkel, J. Ilaš, *Cancers* **2021**, *13*, 3237.
42. N. Karaoun, A. K. A. Renfrew, *Chem. Commun.* (Cambridge, U. K.) **2015**, *51*, 14038–14041.
43. A. Zamora, C. A. Denning, D. K. Heidary, E. Wachter, L. A. Nease, J. Ruiz, E. C. Glazer, *Dalton Trans.* **2017**, *46*, 2165–2173.
44. Z. T. Al-Salama, *Drugs Ther. Perspect.* **2021**, *37*, 393–406.
45. S. Hahner, A. Stürmer, M. Fassnacht, R. W. Hartmann, K. Schewe, S. Cochran, M. Zink, A. Schirbel, B. Allolio, *Horm. Metab. Res.* **2010**, *42*, 528–534.
46. D. Havrylyuk, A. C. Hachey, A. Fenton, D. K. Heidary, E. C. Glazer, *Nat. Commun.* **2022**, 13, 3636.
47. A. N. Carrera, M. K. O. Grant, B. N. Zordoky, *Clin. Sci.* **2020**, *134*, 2897–2927.
48. Y.-J. Chun, S. Kim, *Med. Res. Rev.* **2003**, *23* (6), 657–668.
49. P. F. Guengerich, Y. -J. Chun, D. Kim, E. M. J. Gillam, T. Shimada, *Mut. Res./Fundam. Mol. Mech. Mutagen.* **2003**, 523-524, 173–182.
50. A. Li, R. Yadav, J. K. White, M. K. Herroon, B. P. Callahan, I. Podgorski, C. Turro, E. E. Scott, J. J. Kodanko, *Chem. Commun.* **2017**, 53 (26), 3673–3676.
51. N. Toupin, S. J. Steinke, S. Nadella, A. Li, T. N. Rohrabaugh, E. R. Samuels, C. Turro, I. F. Sevrioukova, J. J. Kodanko, *J. Am. Chem. Soc.* **2021**, *143*, 9191–9205.
52. K. E. Thummel, G. R. Wilkinson, *Annu. Rev. Pharmacol. Toxicol.* **1998**, *38*, 389–430.
53. Y. L. Teo, H. K. Ho, A. Chan, *Br. J. Clin. Pharmacol.* **2015**, *79*, 241–253.
54. S. Breslin, M. C. Lowry, L. O'Driscoll, *Br. J. Cancer* **2017**, *116*, 620–625.
55. P. Kaur, A. R. Chamberlin, T. L. Poulos, I. F. Sevrioukova, *J. Med. Chem.* **2016**, *59*, 4210–4220.
56. E. R. Samuels, I. F. Sevrioukova, *Bioorg. Med. Chem.* **2020**, *28* (6), 115349.
57. E. R. Samuels, I. F. Sevrioukova, *Int. J. Mol. Sci.* **2021**, *22*, 852.
58. L. M. Loftus, J. K. White, B. A. Albani, L. Kohler, J. J. Kodanko, R. P. Thummel, K. R. Dunbar, C. Turro, *Chem. - Eur. J.* **2016**, *22*, 3704–3708.

59. M. V. Blagosklonny, S. C. Dixon, W. D. Figg, J. Urol. **2000**, *163*, 1022–1026.
60. E. Meggers, *Chem. Commun.* **2009**, 1001–1010.
61. C. G. Hartinger, N. Metzler-Nolte, P. J. Dyson, *Organometallics* **2012**, *31*, 5677–5685.
62. G. Gasser, N. Metzler-Nolte, *Curr. Opin. Chem. Biol.* **2012**, *16*, 84–91.
63. G. Gasser, I. Ott, N. Metzler-Nolte, *J. Med. Chem.* **2011**, *54*, 3–25.
64. E. J. Anthony, E. M. Bolitho, H. E. Bridgewater, O. W. L. Carter, J. M. Donnelly, C. Imberti, E. C. Lant, F. Lermyte, R. J. Needham, M. Palau, P. J. Sadler, H. Shi, F. -X. Wang, W. -Y. Zhang, Z. Zhang, *Chem. Sci.* **2020**, *11*, 12888–12917.
65. K. D. Mjos, C. Orvig, *Chem. Rev.* **2014**, *114*, 4540–4563.
66. M. Navarro, E. J. Cisneros-Fajardo, T. Lehmann, R. A. Sánchez-Delgado, R. Atencio, P. Silva, R. Lira, J. A. Urbina, *Inorg. Chem.* **2001**, *40*, 6879–6884.
67. M. Navarro, T. Lehmann, E. J. Cisneros-Fajardo, A. Fuentes, R. A. Sanchez-Delgado, P. Silva, J. A. Urbina, *Polyhedron* **2000**, *19*, 2319–2325
68. R. A. Sanchez-Delgado, K. Lazardi, L. Rincon, J. A. Urbina, A. J. Hubert, A. N. Noels, *J. Med. Chem.* **1993**, *36*, 2041–2043.
69. R. A. Sánchez-Delgado, M. Navarro, K. Lazardi, R. Atencio, M. Capparelli, F. Vargas, J. A. Urbina, A. Bouillez, A. F. Noels, D. Masi, *Inorg. Chim. Acta* **1998**, 275–276, 528–540.
70. E. Iniguez, A. Sánchez, M. A. Vasquez, A. Martínez, J. Olivas, A. Sattler, R. A. Sánchez-Delgado, R. A. Maldonado, *J. Biol. Inorg. Chem.* **2013**, *18*, 779–790.
71. R. -X. Yuan, R. -G. Xiong, B. F. Abrahams, G. -H. Lee, S. -M. Peng, C. -M Che, X. -Z You, *J. Chem. Soc., Dalton Trans.* **2001**, 2071–2073.
72. Y. -Z. Tang, M. Zhou, J. Huang, Z. Cao, T. -T. Qi, G. -H. Huang, H. -R. Wen, *Zeitschrift für anorganische und allgemeine Chemie* **2012**, *638*, 372–376.
73. A. Castonguay, C. Doucet, M. Juhas, D. Maysinger, *J. Med. Chem.* **2012**, *55*, 8799–8806.
74. G. Golbaghi, M. M. Haghdoost, D. Yancu, Y. L. de los Santos, N. Doucet, S. A. Patten, J. T. Sanderson, A. Castonguay, *Organometallics* **2019**, *38*, 702–711.
75. G. Golbaghi, I. Pitard, M. Lucas, M. M. Haghdoost, Y. L. de los Santos, N. Doucet, S. A. Patten, J. T. Sanderson, A. Castonguay, *Eur. J. Med. Chem.* **2020**, *188*, 112030.
76. M. T. Q. Tran, E. Furger, R. Alberto, *Org. Biomol. Chem.* **2013**, *11*, 3247.
77. K. Huang, I. W. Bulik, A. A. Martí, *Chem. Commun.* **2012**, *48*, 11760.
78. K. Huang, C. Jiang, A. A. Martí, *J. Phys. Chem. A* **2014**, *118* (45), 10353–10358.
79. A. A. Martí, C. A. Puckett, J. Dyer, N. Stevens, S. Jockusch, J. Ju, J. K. Barton, N. J. Turro, *J. Am. Chem. Soc.* **2007**, *129*, 8680–8681.
80. K. Huang, A. A. Martí, *Anal. Chem.* **2012**, *84*, 8075–8082.
81. A. Saha, Z. Panos, T. Hanna, K. Huang, M. Hernández-Rivera, A. A. Martí, *Angew. Chem., Int. Ed.* **2013**, *52*, 12615–12618.
82. T. L. Poulos, B. C. Finzel, A. J. Howard, *J. Mol. Biol.* **1987**, *195*, 687–700.
83. A. Greule, J. E. Stok, J. J. De Voss, M. J. Cryle, *Nat. Prod. Rep.* **2018**, *35*, 757–791.
84. T. Kamachi, K. A. Yoshizawa, *J. Am. Chem. Soc.* **2003**, *125*, 4652–4661.
85. P. Urban, T. Lautier, D. Pompon, G. Truan, *Int. J. Mol. Sci.* **2018**, 19, 1617.
86. A. R. Dunn, I. J. Dmochowski, A. M. Bilwes, H. B. Gray, B. R. Crane, *Proc. Natl. Acad. Sci. U.S.A.* **2001**, *98*, 12420–12425.
87. I. J. Dmochowski, B. R. Crane, J. J. Wilker, Winkler, H. B. Gray, *Proc. Natl. Acad. Sci. U.S.A.* **1999**, *96*, 12987–12990.
88. A. -M. A. Hays, A. R. Dunn, R. Chiu, H. B. Gray, C. D. Stout, D. B. Goodin, *J. Mol. Biol.* **2004**, *344*, 455–469.
89. A. R. Dunn, A. -M. A. Hays, D. B. Goodin, C. D. Stout, R. Chiu, J. R. Winkler, H. B. Gray, *J. Am. Chem. Soc.* **2002**, *124*, 10254–10255.

90. M. Denison, S. J. Steinke, A. Majeed, C. Turro, T. A. Kocarek, I. F. Sevrioukova, J. J. Kodanko, *Inorg. Chem.* **2022**, *61*, 13673–13677.
91. M. Denison, J. J. Ahrens, M. N. Dunbar, H. Warmahaye, A. Majeed, C. Turro, T. A. Kocarek, I. F. Sevrioukova, J. J. Kodanko, *Inorg. Chem.* **2023**, *62*, 3305–3320.
92. T. Yoshihara, S. Murayama, T. Masuda, T. Kikuchi, K. Yoshida, M. Hosaka, S. Tobita, *J. Photochem. Photobiol. A* **2015**, *299*, 172–182.
93. K. Koren, R. I. Dmitriev, S. M. Borisov, D. B. Papkovsky, I. Klimant, *Chembiochem* **2012**, *13*, 1184–1190.
94. K.Y. Zhang, T. Zhang, H. Wei, Q. Wu, S. Liu, Q. Zhao, W. Huang, *Chem. Sci.* **2018**, *9*, 7236–7240.
95. K. Y. Zhang, P. Gao, G. Sun, T. Zhang, X. Li, S. Liu, Q. Zhao, K. K. -W. Lo, W. Huang, *J. Am. Chem. Soc.* **2018**, *140*, 7827–7834.
96. Y. Dai, Z. Zhan, L. Chai, L. Zhang, Q. Guo, K. Zhang, Y. Lv, *Anal. Chem.* **2021**, *93*, 4628–4634.
97. S. P. -Y. Li, J. Shum, K. K. -W. Lo, *Dalton Trans.* **2019**, *48*, 9692–9702.
98. L. Xiong, Q. Zhao, H. Chen, Y. Wu, Z. Dong, Z. Zhou, F. Li, *Inorg. Chem.* **2010**, *49*, 6402–6408.
99. Y. Li, Y. Wu, L. Chen, H. Zeng, X. Chen, W. Lun, X. Fan, W. -Y. A. Wong, *J. Mater. Chem. B* **2019**, *7*, 7612–7618.

5 Heme-Based Therapeutics

Elmira Alipour
Department of Physics
Wake Forest University
Winston-Salem, North Carolina 27109, USA
alipe17@wfu.edu

Mark T. Gladwin
Department of Medicine
University of Maryland School of Medicine
Baltimore, Maryland 21201, USA
MGladwin@som.umaryland.edu

Daniel B. Kim-Shapiro
Department of Physics
Wake Forest University
Winston-Salem, North Carolina 27109, USA
shapiro@wfu.edu

CONTENTS

DOI: 10.1201/9781003361756-5

ABSTRACT

Heme is a ubiquitous cofactor used in a variety of proteins including hemoglobin, myoglobin, nitric oxide synthase, soluble guanylyl cyclase, cytochrome c, and
cytochrome c oxidase. On the other hand, free heme can facilitate various deleterious redox reactions via activation of danger-associated molecular pattern signaling
pathways and the inflammasome. Given the multitude of functions of heme proteins
and the potential toxicity of free heme, it is no wonder that the use of heme-containing proteins as well as heme scavenger molecules has been developed for therapeutic use. In this chapter, we review these developments, including hemoglobin-based
oxygen carriers for use as "blood substitutes," heme-globins for use as antidotes for
carbon monoxide poisoning, and S-nitroso hemoglobin for use in a variety of conditions. We also describe nitrite-based therapies for cardiovascular diseases that rely
on nitrite reactions with hemoglobin. Finally, we review work on NO ferroheme
(nitric oxide bound to a ferrous heme), related to recent discoveries on its chemistry
of formation and vascular effects.

KEYWORDS

Heme; Hemoglobin; Blood Substitutes; Nitric Oxide; Nitrite; Carbon
Monoxide

1   INTRODUCTION

Heme is a planar molecule consisting of protoporphyrin IX with an iron atom
coordinated to the four pyrole rings. The iron is usually in the ferrous ($+2$), ferric
($+3$), or sometimes ferryl ($+4$) form (Figure 1). The term "heme" is often used to
describe the ferrous form, while "hemin" is used to describe the ferric form, but
we will simply use the term heme to include all iron oxidation states. Heme is a
common prosthetic group found in many proteins, including hemoglobin (Hb),
myoglobin, nitric oxide synthase (NOS), soluble guanylyl cyclase (sGC), cytochrome c, and cytochrome c oxidase. Its functions include oxygen transport and
storage, bioenergetics, and many others. In addition to its functions while bound
to these and other proteins, it is now appreciated that heme functions as a signaling molecule [1–5]. Heme has been described as a DAMP (danger-associated
molecular pattern) molecule [2,5] promoting inflammation through interactions

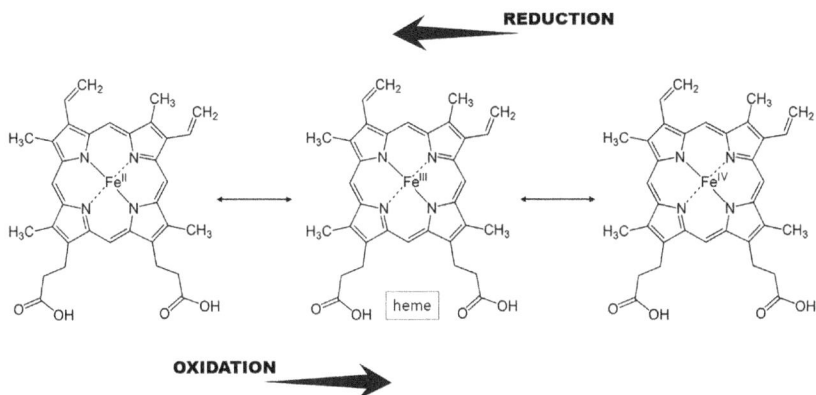

FIGURE 1 Heme. The heme is shown in its various oxidation states.

with TL4 (toll-like receptors) [2]. In addition, labile and exchangeable heme has been shown to bind various heme-responsive sensors, influencing many biological functions, including transcription, protein degradation, and ion transport [1].

In this chapter, we review examples of how heme-containing proteins have been developed for therapeutic use. We start with hemoglobin-based oxygen carriers (HBOCs). Use of cell-free hemoglobin or a modified form of this oxygen-carrying molecule as a blood substitute has been actively pursued for about 100 years [6]. This is because human donor red blood cells require cold storage, antigen matching, and pathogen testing. Sometimes, stored blood is in short supply, while other times, stored blood leads to transfusion reactions that cannot be properly matched to the recipient. In addition, there are situations, such as on the battlefield, where stored blood availability is limited. Much work has been done developing HBOCs with some success.

We next turn to the use of several heme proteins and their variants as an antidote for carbon monoxide (CO) poisoning. CO binds to hemoglobin about 200 times more strongly than oxygen. The CO also binds to cytochrome c oxidase, shutting down oxidative phosphorylation, which leads to substantial morbidity and mortality. The heme-protein–based strategy is to develop a product that binds CO tighter than hemoglobin so that it can be administered as a point-of-care therapy. Use of nitrite is also discussed as a means to deliver NO activity. In this chapter, when we refer to nitrite and nitrate, we mean inorganic forms (as opposed to organic nitrates). It is worth noting that sodium nitrite is Food and Drug Administration–approved as a therapy for cyanide poisoning. In this application, nitrite is administered in sufficient quantities to oxidize hemoglobin to the ferric, methemoglobin form, which tightly binds cyanide, sparing cytochrome oxidase and reducing toxicity. In this chapter, we focus on other developing therapeutics using nitrite. Another product that we explore is the use of S-nitrosated hemoglobin (SNO-Hb) to deliver NO activity. This product has been explored for a variety of indications. Finally, we discuss the use of NO ferroheme to deliver NO activity, an area of recent intense interest.

2   HEMOGLOBIN-BASED OXYGEN CARRIERS

2.1   Need and History of Hemoglobin-Based Oxygen Carriers (HBOCs)

In the United States, about 29,000 units of stored red blood cells are needed for transfusions every day. These life-saving transfusions replenish the blood's oxygen transport capacity in a variety of conditions, including trauma, anemic diseases such as sickle cell disease and malaria, and during surgeries. However, the requirement for large amounts of stored blood makes it difficult to meet demand, and it sometimes falls short. There have been critical shortages at certain times across the globe [6]. Several factors exacerbate the potential for shortages in our blood supply. Packed red blood cells have a finite shelf life of 42 days in the United States. The red blood cells must be stored at low temperatures. Viruses present in the blood of the donor, such as HIV or hepatitis, can limit supply. Antigen matching can be difficult, especially for certain individuals that require chronic transfusions and develop alloimmunization. Finally, the need for red blood cells can be especially important on the battlefield in situations where it is hard to deliver a viable product. Thus, there is a desire or, in fact, a need to develop a product that can substitute for the oxygen-delivering capacity of red blood cell-encapsulated hemoglobin without these limitations.

The exploration of the use of extracellular hemoglobin as a blood substitute has been undertaken since at least the 1930s [6,7]. Early studies were associated with substantial toxicity, including hypertension, renal failure, cardiac issues, and the excretion of large amounts of hemoglobin [6,7]. Despite enormous public and private efforts, success has been limited, and no HBOCs have been approved for human use by the FDA or European Medicines Agency (EMA) [8]. However, trials are ongoing, and human use has been approved in some parts of the world.

2.2   Challenges in Developing HBOCs

The main issues that have been associated with various HBOCs are related to poor oxygen delivery, nitric oxide (NO) scavenging, and oxidative damage (Figure 2). Red blood cells have evolved to be ideal oxygen delivery agents that minimize NO scavenging and oxidative damage. Progress has been made, but sometimes partially overcoming one challenge makes another one worse.

Hemoglobin is a tetramer with two alpha and two beta subunits. Each subunit contains a heme group that can bind one oxygen molecule, so that one hemoglobin tetramer can bind four oxygen molecules. Efficient delivery of oxygen by hemoglobin is made possible by cooperative oxygen binding and release. Cooperativity allows hemoglobin to be fully bound to oxygen in the lungs and then released in the tissues. Cooperative binding is where, after binding the first oxygen, the binding of subsequent oxygen molecules by hemoglobin becomes easier. This is also true in the release of oxygen. Cooperativity can be explained by the Mond-Wyman-Changeux (MWC) or MWC-Perutz two-state model [9,10].

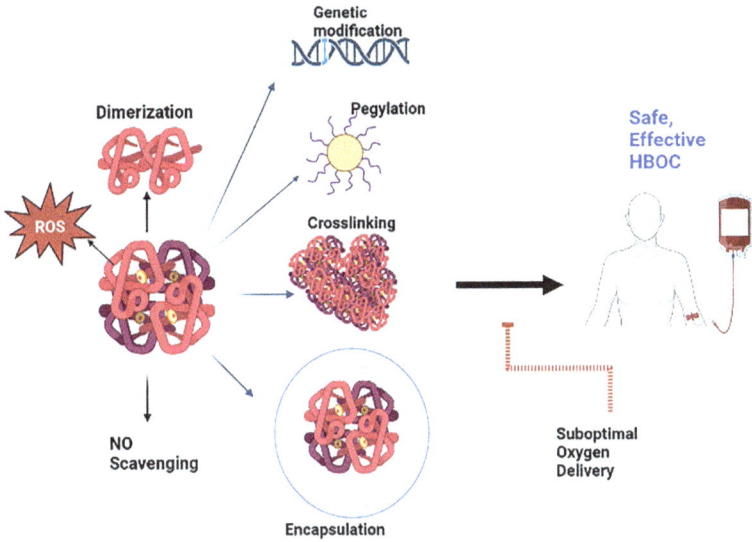

FIGURE 2 HBOC development. Issues are shown associated with the development of a viable HBOC, including oxidative stress due to reactive oxygen species (ROS), dimerization, which exacerbates oxidative stress, and NO scavenging. General approaches to overcome these obstacles are shown, including genetic modification, pegylation, crosslinking (representing both inter- and intra-molecular crosslinking), and encapsulation in membrane vesicles. Another obstacle that persists is that many developments that overcome some obstacles end up with a product that has poor oxygen delivery characteristics, at least compared to native red cell hemoglobin (this figure was made using Biorender (Biorender.com)).

The two states include the high oxygen affinity R-state and the low oxygen affinity T-state, and they differ in their quaternary structure. When a hemoglobin molecule has no oxygen bound, it will be in the T-state. After two to three oxygen molecules bind, the tetramer undergoes a conformational change to the R-state. This allosteric transition (where binding at one heme affects binding affinity at other hemes) makes it so that the hemoglobin favors being in the R-state at the lungs so that it binds the maximum amount of oxygen and the hemoglobin molecule favors being in the T-state in conditions of relatively low oxygen tension like the tissues so that it releases the oxygen.

A major challenge in developing an HBOC is to make one that can mimic the oxygen-binding properties of hemoglobin in the red blood cell. Inside the red blood cell, hemoglobin is bound to 2,3-diphosphoglycerate (DPG), which reduces the affinity of the hemoglobin by stabilizing the T-state and facilitating oxygen delivery. In plasma, without DPG, oxygen delivery by hemoglobin is impaired. As described above, efficient oxygen delivery is dependent on the function of the hemoglobin tetramer. However, hemoglobin dimerizes into two alpha-beta dimers with a dissociation constant of about one micromolar. Thus, while inside the red blood cell (where there is about 20 millimolar hemoglobin in heme), only a very small percentage is dimers, but with 100 micromolar extracellular hemoglobin, about 10% of the heme will be in hemoglobin dimers. NO scavenging (discussed below) limits how much cell-free hemoglobin can be present. The dimers cannot bind oxygen cooperatively and bind oxygen with an affinity similar to R-state hemoglobin. Thus, cell-free hemoglobin in plasma has a higher affinity for oxygen than in red blood cells. Investigators have suggested that the higher affinity leads to premature oxygen unloading and that this contributes to vasoconstriction in tissues [11].

Nitric oxide is an important signaling molecule that affects vasodilation to increase blood flow, decreases platelet activation and adhesion of circulating blood cells to the endothelial walls of the blood vessel, and can act as an anti-inflammatory agent [12]. Nitric oxide is produced in the endothelial cells surrounding blood vessels by an enzyme called NOS. The NO must then diffuse from the endothelium to the smooth muscles, where it binds to sGC, which increases cyclic guanosine monophosphate (cGMP) and signals muscle relaxation that increases blood flow. However, NO reacts with oxygenated hemoglobin at near diffusion-limited rates $(6-8 \times 10^7 \text{ M}^{-1}\text{s}^{-1})$, a process deemed dioxygenation [13].

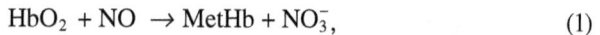

$$HbO_2 + NO \rightarrow MetHb + NO_3^-, \tag{1}$$

where HbO_2 is oxygenated hemoglobin, MetHb is methemoglobin, which is when the heme iron is oxidized to +3, and NO_3^- is nitrate. The presence of millimolar amounts of oxygenated hemoglobin immediately adjacent to where it is made begs the question of how NO can effectively signal during dioxygenation [14].

Importantly, encapsulation of hemoglobin inside the red blood cell limits the rate of NO dioxygenation by several mechanisms, including (1) a cell-free zone in which red blood cells tend to flow toward the middle of the blood vessel, leaving a zone next to the endothelia so that NO dioxygenation is lessened; (2) rate limitations due to diffusion, also called the unstirred layer, whereby the rate of NO scavenging is limited by the time it takes for the NO to diffuse to the red blood cell; and possibly (3) rate limitations due to the NO needing to diffuse across the membrane [15]. Even in the absence of the cell-free zone, for example, as measured by stopped-flow absorption, the rate of NO reaction with oxygenated hemoglobin in the red blood cell can be as slow as 1,000 times slower than with cell-free hemoglobin [16,17]. However, at more physiological hematocrits where the high red cell mass creates a significant surface area for NO diffusion and reaction with intracellular hemoglobin, cell-free hemoglobin still reacts with NO about 50 (as opposed to 1,000) times faster than red blood cell-encapsulated hemoglobin [17]. In any case, due to the faster NO scavenging, cell-free hemoglobin can greatly reduce NO bioavailability, which increases blood pressure; some HBOCs have been observed to increase mean arterial blood pressure by as much as 30 mm Hg [7]. In addition, due to their small size, cell-free hemoglobin, and particularly hemoglobin dimers, can extravasate into the interstitial space between the endothelium and smooth muscle, and this greatly exacerbates NO scavenging [18].

Heme iron is the source of a variety of redox chemical reactions [19–21]. Autoxidation of oxygenated hemoglobin produces methemoglobin and superoxide.

$$HbO_2 \rightarrow MetHb + O_2^-, \qquad (2)$$

The superoxide rapidly dismutates into the reactive oxygen species (ROS) hydrogen peroxide. Hydrogen peroxide can subsequently react with either oxidized or reduced hemoglobin to make ferryl species that perpetuate the formation of ROS, causing oxidative damage and, under certain circumstances, leading to inflammatory responses. In addition, methemoglobin can lose its heme groups, which in turn can produce non-transferrin–bound iron, and these also further exacerbate ROS production and oxidative damage.

The red blood cell contains several systems that reduce oxidative damage that are not available in the plasma. Methemoglobin reductase converts methemoglobin back to the reduced hemoglobin species. Superoxide dismutase catalyzes the dismutation of superoxide into water and hydrogen peroxide. Catalase decomposes hydrogen peroxide into water and oxygen. Peroxiredoxin also produces water from hydrogen peroxide, as does glutathione peroxidase. Glutathione (GSH) is highly abundant in red blood cells (3–5 mM), which itself offers protection against oxidative stress, while reduced thiol content in plasma is much lower (<1 mM, mostly in albumin [22]).

2.3   APPROACHES EMPLOYED TO OVERCOME CHALLENGES ENCOUNTERED IN DEVELOPING HBOCS

Figure 2 depicts some general strategies used to overcome challenges related to HBOC toxicity. Most, if not all, efforts to modulate the oxygen-binding properties of HBOCs have been to lower their oxygen affinity because cell-free hemoglobin dimerizes and loses DPG, causing oxygen to bind too tightly for efficient delivery. One approach has been to employ pyridoxal phosphate as a DPG mimetic, which stabilizes the T-state [7]. Bovine hemoglobin naturally has a low oxygen affinity compared to humans, binds chloride tightly (which stabilizes the T-state), and has been used in a glutaraldehyde polymerized form to make a product called Hemopure that is authorized for compassionate use for people who refuse normal transfusions and approved for human use in South Africa and Russia [7,8]. Pegylation (conjugation with polyethylene glycol) of hemoglobin has been studied extensively and led to several products where the oxygen affinity depends on where the pegylation occurs in the hemoglobin molecule [8]. Whether the hemoglobin is modified through inter- or intra-molecular crosslinking under oxygenated or deoxygenated conditions greatly influences its oxygen affinity [8]. In addition, the oxygen affinity has been controlled through mutations in the distal heme pocket [7].

A key strategy employed to reduce NO scavenging is to prevent tetramer dimerization and increase the size of the HBOC so that it does not extravasate. Both intra- and inter-molecular crosslinking accomplishes this. In addition, encapsulation of hemoglobin in membrane vesicles also greatly reduces the rate of NO scavenging, partially due to rate-limiting diffusion to the vesicle [23]. However, given the relatively small size of these membrane vesicles compared to red blood cells, they still likely enter the cell-free zone, similarly to natural red cell microparticles [24]. Coating the HBOC with polyethylene glycol polymers increases the size of the Hb substantially, and measured effects on hypertension suggest that the larger the HBOC, the less extravasation and the less NO scavenging [25]. Thus, polymerized HBOCs have less of an effect on blood pressure than intra-molecular cross-linked HBOCs [7]. Another strategy has been to express modified hemoglobins that, through strategic amino acid substitutions, reduce the rate of NO dioxygenation by up to about 20-fold, with corresponding decreases in hypertensive effects [7].

When employed at therapeutic concentrations, many cross-linked HBOCs undergo autoxidation (Equation 2) faster than normal adult hemoglobin, so oxidative damage is an issue [7]. A challenge in developing optimal HBOCs is that autoxidation is most efficient when the hemoglobin is partially oxygenated, but HBOCs that have too high oxygen affinity do not efficiently deliver oxygen. An effective strategy is to engineer hemoglobin variants that have reduced rates of autoxidation [7]. Protein engineering has also been used to develop HBOCs that minimize heme loss (which also exacerbates oxidative stress), but success has been limited, with no product performing better than native normal adult hemoglobin [7].

2.4   CURRENT STATE AND FUTURE OUTLOOK

Initially, the development of HBOCs as a blood substitute to be used in place of transfusion may have been thought to be a straight-forward, easy task. However, when one examines the history of product development by several companies, one observes that a majority of products have failed, several after phase III clinical trials [6]. It should be noted that in addition to having favorable oxygen delivery properties, minimal NO scavenging, and limited oxidative stress, it must be practical to produce sufficient quantities of a viable HBOC. A few products have, at least partially, achieved these goals. Hemopure (also now developed as HBOC-201), a glutaraldehyde polymerized bovine hemoglobin product, has been approved for human use in South Africa and Russia [6,8]. A similar product made by the same company (Biopure), called Oxyglobin, is approved for animal use in the United States [6]. Hemopure, along with Sanguinate, which is a pegylated bovine hemoglobin product, are approved for compassionate use in cases where blood transfusions are refused or cannot be carried out [8]. There are also several HBOCs that are undergoing further development and clinical trials. Hemoact is a hemoglobin conjugated to albumin that has a favorable oxygen affinity and has successfully been tested in animals [8,26]. Erythromer is a membrane encapsulated product that includes DPG inside the 0.15 µm vesicle that can also be lyophilized and has favorable oxygen-binding properties and minimal NO scavenging [26,27]. In addition, HBOCs have, in some cases, been repurposed. Several products are being developed or are in current use to help preserve organs for tissue transplantation, including Hemopure and HemO2life, a product derived from a marine worm [6,8,28]. Another pegylated HBOC, MP4, has been explored as an agent for CO delivery [8,29].

Despite many challenges, one notes that progress has been made, but there is still much work to do in order to achieve a viable blood product. Given the enormous benefits of such a product, we suggest that this work is worthwhile.

3   CARBON MONOXIDE ANTIDOTES

3.1   CARBON MONOXIDE POISONING

Per the Centers for Disease Control and Prevention, after misuse and abusive use of analgesic drugs, CO is the leading cause of non-drug–related human poisoning illnesses and deaths in the United States every year. Chemical substances such as cleaning agents, pesticides, and personal care products are other examples of the top ten causes of poisoning deaths. CO is an odorless, tasteless, and colorless gas, which is hence named the "silent killer." Victims of this poisoning can become sick or die before realizing they are exposed. Examples of CO sources are burning charcoal and wood (fireplace), grills, gas stoves and ovens, lanterns, motor vehicle exhausts, furnaces, kerosene heaters, tobacco smoke, and more. High concentrations of enclosed and indoor CO from such sources may lead to death in less than a few minutes as CO gas is inhaled and enters the lungs. Centers for Disease Control and Prevention statistics show that approximately 500 people die in the United States from over 100,000 annual emergency visits for accidental CO poisoning (https://www.cdc.gov/co/default.htm). The symptoms of CO poisoning can be misleading and difficult to identify. Flu-like early symptoms such as headache, fatigue, dizziness, nausea, vomiting, and chest pain may progress to irritability, impaired coordination, and eventually loss of consciousness [30]. As lungs absorb and transport CO to the bloodstream, it binds to ferrous iron(II) heme proteins like myoglobin in muscles or hemoglobin molecules, as it has 250 times higher affinity than oxygen for ferrous heme. Upon CO binding, any or all oxygen-binding sites of hemoglobin can be occupied by CO molecules [31–33]. In addition, partial binding of CO to hemoglobin can lock it in the R-state and thereby inhibit oxygen delivery.

Complex IV (COX), the final protein complex of the electron transport chain, is located in the inner mitochondrial membrane. It transports electrons from cytochrome c, the electron carrier, and reduces O_2 to water molecules. CO poisoning inhibits oxidative phosphorylation, proton transportation, and oxygen reduction to H_2O and shuts off the respiratory chain by blocking the last electron transport in cytochrome c oxidase, similar to the effects of cyanide and azide. Inhibited mitochondrial respiration, poisoned mitochondria, and elevated toxic levels of hemoglobin-bound carbon monoxide (COHb) cause mortality [32].

3.2   TREATING CO POISONING

Despite being a significant cause of human morbidity, CO poisoning does not have any existing or approved antidotal therapy up to date that has reached phase III clinical trials; thus, there are no effective medical interventions to neutralize CO *in vivo* [31,34]. This gas poisoning is currently treated by hyperbaric or normobaric oxygen inhalation therapy to increase plasma-O_2 saturation and the conversion of carboxy-hemoglobin and carboxymyoglobin to hemoglobin and myoglobin [35]. Additionally, these current therapies are not ideal and have both short- and long-term negative effects, such as low efficacy of oxygen therapy due to the delay between the official diagnostics and initiating therapy, oxygen toxicity, pulmonary edema and lung damage, hemorrhage, inner-ear barotraumas, nitrogen emboli, risk of seizure, and more [35,36]. One possible resolution that has been explored more recently is fast CO removal through the kidneys. In this method, a molecule with high affinity for CO captures CO from hemoglobin in red blood cells and clears out poisoning CO molecules from blood and tissues [31,32,37–41]. This strategy is depicted in Figure 3.

In one recent study, a novel hemoprotein-based CO scavenging therapy was developed using an engineered variant of human neuroglobin (Ngb-H64Q-CCC) [32]. This protein, with a 500-fold higher affinity toward CO than that of hemoglobin, was tested in a severe CO-poisoned rat model and was able to reverse CO-induced hypotension, recover tissue respiration and cytochrome c oxidase activity, and improve survival to 87.5%, compared to less than 10% survival in control animals receiving intravenous fluid resuscitation only [32].

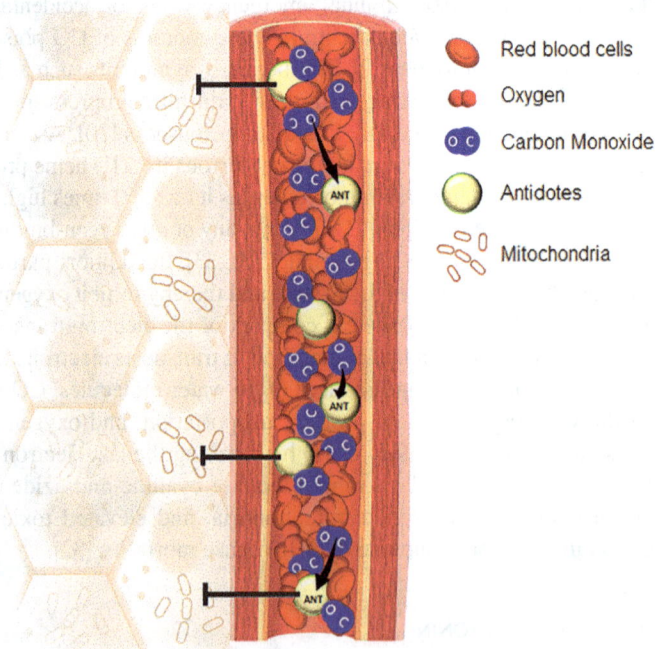

Legend:
- Red blood cells
- Oxygen
- Carbon Monoxide
- Antidotes
- Mitochondria

FIGURE 3   A proposed antidote strategy to treat CO poisoning. The antidote is infused into the blood, where it captures CO from red blood cells, preventing CO from diffusing into tissue, where it can interfere with mitochondrial respiration.

Readily available hemoproteins, stripped hemoglobin, and N-ethylmaleimide bound to hemoglobin, which stabilize the R-state (StHb and NEMHb), were investigated in another research study on a rat model to control blood pressure and heart rate, preventing hemodynamic collapse after CO exposure. Faster recombination rates and comparable dissociation rates compared to R-state hemoglobin, along with high "M values" (the binding affinity to CO compared to oxygen), which are the main criteria for finding suitable antidotes, resulted in these two proteins being considerable effective point-of-care options [38].

Aligned with finding molecules with high affinity toward CO, hemoCDs, the water-soluble, porphyrin-containing molecules solubilized by two CycloDextrin ligands, have also been studied [42]. In order to overcome simultaneous poisoning with CO and hydrogen cyanide, another group suggested hemoCD-Twins as a great prospective ready-to-use antidote against fire gas poisoning [34].

3.3 Antidotal Therapy Prospect

CO, which is the most common non-drug human poison, lacks clinical methods of therapy beyond increasing public awareness and efforts made for public safety improvement. The goal is to develop and introduce a point-of-care antidote that could potentially be infused immediately on site into the victims of CO poisoning. Future developments may include non-pharmacologic therapies or pharmacologic antidotes to reverse carboxyhemoglobin formations in red blood cells and to scavenge CO molecules. Further studies are necessary not only to investigate more hemoprotein-based therapeutic candidates but also to test the findings in next phase trials on large mammals and humans.

Another prospective study is to test the efficacy and influence of superoxide dismutase, catalase, and other related ROS as adjuvants to hemoCD-Twins with the aim of granting a worldwide used gas poisoning antidote [31,34]. In addition, current studies are examining mutants of neuroglobins, cytoglobins, and various bacterial proteins, as they have considerably higher CO association rates compared to hemoglobin, supported by successful outcomes in past research [32,38].

4 NITRITE

4.1 Nitrite Physiology

While some human studies observed no arterial-venous gradients for SNO-Hb, arterial levels of nitrosyl hemoglobin were measured to be higher than venous levels, as were nitrite levels, including at baseline, after NO inhalation, and when inhibiting NOS, and these gradients were potentiated during exercise [43,44]. The gradients suggest the delivery of NO activity to tissue. Although one study had suggested that nitrite is inert in human physiology [45], subsequent human studies showed that nitrite is a potent vasodilator and that its action is potentiated with exercise and under hypoxic conditions [46,47]. Nitrite reacts with deoxygenated hemoglobin to form NO [48,49].

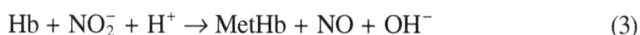

$$Hb + NO_2^- + H^+ \rightarrow MetHb + NO + OH^- \tag{3}$$

where MetHb is the ferric form of the heme and Hb represents a vacant (deoxygenated) heme in hemoglobin. These findings led to the proposal that hemoglobin reduces nitrite to NO upon partial deoxygenation so that it is both the sensor for low oxygen and the producer of NO activity when it is needed [46]. As seen in Equation 3, reduction of nitrite by deoxyhemoglobin is favored at lower pH, and the notion of non-enzymatic acidic reduction of nitrite to NO has also been suggested by others [50,51]. Adding to the paradigm that hemoglobin functions to deliver NO to hypoxic tissues, nitrite reduction by hemoglobin was observed to be under allosteric control, so that the rate of nitrite reduction is balanced by the availability of deoxygenated hemes and faster intrinsic reduction by R-state hemoglobin compared to T-sate, resulting in maximal NO production near the hemoglobin p50 [52,53].

The biggest challenge to the nitrite hemoglobin hypothesis is that NO produced within the red blood cell should be rapidly scavenged by oxygenated hemoglobin under physiological conditions through dioxygenation (Equation 2). Several possible mechanisms have been proposed through which NO activity could be exported following nitrite bioactivation by red blood cells, including compartmentalization within the red blood cell [54] and the formation of intermediate species including nitrosothiols, N_2O_3, and others [55–59]. Regardless of the mechanism by which nitrite is bioactivated by red blood cells, there is substantial evidence from a variety of experiments that nitrite production of NO activity is dependent on red blood cells. Several different types of experiments have been conducted where the effects of NO upon nitrite addition are either potentiated or even completely dependent on the presence of red blood cells. Work from the Patel lab has shown that relaxation of aortic ring preparations by nitrite is greatly potentiated by the presence of red blood cells, especially under hypoxic conditions [46,60]. This potentiation in activity by red blood cells was also observed with nitrite-dependent inhibition of mitochondrial respiration [60,61]. Similarly, whereas nitrite has no activity regarding inhibition of platelet activation in the absence of red blood cells, when red blood cells are present, physiologically relevant concentrations of nitrite inhibit platelet aggregation and activation [58,62]. All of these actions are known to involve canonical NO signaling, thereby strongly supporting the proposal that red blood cell hemoglobin bioactivates nitrite, producing NO bioactivity.

4.2   NITRITE THERAPEUTICS

The maximal tolerable dose for nitrite infusions in healthy human volunteers was established, even for long-term infusions with toxicity monitoring for hypotension and methemoglobin formation [63]. Nitrite infusion studies have been conducted in animals and/or humans to examine treatments for a variety of conditions, including prevention of delayed cerebral vasospasm after subarachnoid hemorrhage [64], protection against ischemic-reperfusion injury [65,66], and sickle cell disease [67]. In a murine study of nitrite administration, improvements were observed in lowering hemolysis and decreasing adhesion of lymphocytes and platelets to the endothelium [68]. Inhaled nitrite has also been studied as a therapeutic for pulmonary hypertension and/or heart failure with preserved ejection fraction [69].

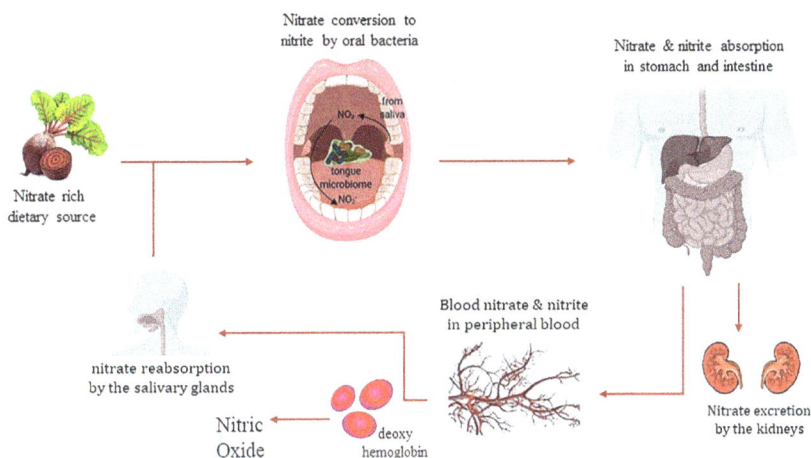

FIGURE 4 Nitrate-Nitrite-NO cycle. Nitrate, which is abundant in foods like beetroot, is partially reduced by oral bacteria to nitrite. Nitrate and nitrite then enter the blood stream through the digestive system. Nitrite is reduced to nitric oxide by hemoglobin. Remaining nitrate (not excreted by the kidneys) is taken up by the salivary glands into the oral cavity, so the cycle continues (adapted from Lundberg et al. [71], Ma et al. [111], and Grant and Jonsson [112]).

In addition to infusing and inhaling nitrite, it can also be administered orally, and studies have been conducted to examine its efficacy in treating various conditions, for example, hypertension and metabolic syndrome [70]. An attractive way to increase plasma nitrite is through oral intake of dietary nitrate, for example, through drinking high-nitrate beetroot juice. Use of dietary nitrate is based on the nitrate-nitrite-NO cycle [71]. Nitrate is partially reduced to nitrite by oral bacteria. Nitrate and nitrite are taken up from the digestive system to the blood, where nitrite can deliver NO activity. Importantly, the remaining nitrate is taken back up into the oral cavity by the salivary glands, where the concentrated nitrate is again partially reduced by nitrite. In this way, the half-life of nitrate is on the order of 6 hours, and someone can drink beetroot juice in the morning and have elevated plasma nitrite all day long. This "Nitrate-Nitrite-NO" cycle is depicted in Figure 4. Dietary nitrate has been shown to have positive effects in several clinical trials, including cerebral blood flow and brain connectivity [72,73], chronic obstructive pulmonary disease [74], heart failure and preserved ejection fraction [75,76], platelet activation [77], vascular function [78], peripheral artery disease [79–81], and hypertension [82]. Dietary nitrate has been of interest as a method to improve exercise performance in healthy individuals and athletes [83–86].

4.3 CHALLENGES WITH NITRITE THERAPEUTICS

Despite all of the work conducted as referred to above, none has resulted in FDA approval for the use of nitrite or nitrate for any conditions. The precise mechanism of how NO activity is exported from the red blood cell remains to be solved. However, due to the fact that the efficacy of other NO donors is blunted or abrogated by the presence of red blood cells (presumably through deoxygenation) (Equation 2), while nitrite requires the presence of red blood cells for bioactivation [68], nitrite may be the best NO donor to use in blood. Work is continuing both at the basic science level and in clinical studies. For example, there is currently a phase III clinical trial underway (NCT05624125) examining if daily intake of nitrate-rich beetroot juice improves 6-minute walk tests in patients with peripheral artery disease.

5   S-NITROSOHEMOGLOBIN (SNO-Hb)

5.1   THE SNO-Hb HYPOTHESIS

The SNO-Hb hypothesis has been developed by Stamler and colleagues (Figure 5, adapted from [87,88]). SNO-Hb is formed by S-nitrosation of the β93 cysteine, and S-nitrosation (also referred to as nitrosylation in analogy to protein phosphorylation) occurs preferentially in R-state hemoglobin. Both low- and high-molecular weight nitrosothiols preserve NO activity because they avoid a rapid reaction with oxygenated hemoglobin (Equation 1). The SNO-Hb hypothesis involves an allosterically controlled, hemoglobin-mediated delivery of NO activity to increase blood flow in hypoxic tissue (where it is needed). In this model, SNO-Hb is formed preferentially under relatively high oxygen tension at the lungs when the hemoglobin is in the R-state, and upon deoxygenation and transition to the T-state,

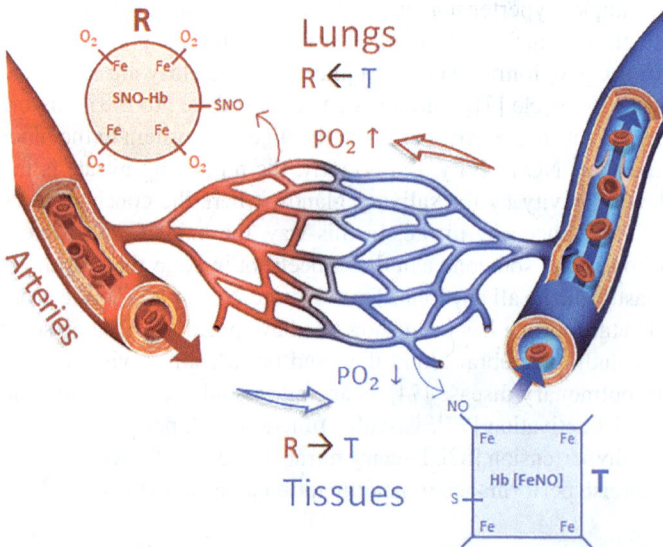

FIGURE 5   The SNO-Hb hypothesis. Hemoglobin is S-nitrosated at the lungs, with hemoglobin in the R-state. Upon transport to the tissues, hemoglobin undergoes a change to the T-state, where nitrosation at the β93 cysteine is disfavored and NO binds to the heme while NO activity is also exported from red blood cells (adapted from McMahon et al. [88]).

the NO (or NO$^+$) is released from the β93 cysteine and exported from the red blood cell through trans-nitrosation reactions involving low molecular weight thiols like GSH and cysteine [88]. In addition, some of the NO on the β93 cysteine is transferred to the heme, forming iron nitrosyl hemoglobin. Upon reoxygenation, NO on the heme is transferred back to the β93 cysteine [88]. The transfer of NO from heme to β93 cysteine was supported by data presented on measured species in venous and arterial blood from human subjects [88]. The ability of SNO-Hb to target NO delivery to areas of the body that need it (hypoxia) and to preserve NO activity through formation of nitrosothiols was suggested to play important roles in normal physiology and could be employed for therapeutic purposes [87,88].

5.2 SNO-Hb THERAPEUTICS

Given its proposed important role in normal physiology, it is no surprise that dysfunctions in SNO-Hb function have been suggested to play important roles in the pathology of several diseases and pathological conditions. These include sickle cell disease, where the allosterically controlled intra-molecular transfer between heme and β93 cysteine is reported to be impaired in the sickle cell hemoglobin along with export of NO activity from the red blood cell [89]. In addition, hypoxia is suggested to lead to an imbalance in the amounts of iron, nitrosyl hemoglobin, and SNO-Hb that contributes to pulmonary hypertension [90]. Loss of SNO-Hb has also been suggested to be an important aspect of the blood "storage lesion," whereby red blood cells stored for transfusion lose their functional capacity [91].

In a small study, inhalation of ethyl nitrite (1.5–70 ppm) resulted in substantial increases in SNO-Hb, which decreased pulmonary arterial pressure and pulmonary vascular resistance in a dose-dependent manner in patients with pulmonary hypertension [90]. Stamler and colleagues also studied the effects of SNO-Hb repletion in stored blood upon transfusion in mice, rats, and sheep [92]. The SNO-Hb–repleted stored blood performed better than control in measurements in all models. In the sheep model, where SNO-Hb was formed by exposure to ethyl nitrite, oxygen delivery was improved, and renal blood flow and kidney function that were negatively affected upon transfusion of control stored blood were not affected by SNO-Hb–repleted stored blood [92].

5.3 ISSUES RELATED TO SNO-Hb

The notion that hemoglobin transports not only oxygen and carbon dioxide but also NO is attractive. However, several reports have challenged various aspects of the SNO-Hb hypothesis, including several from the authors of this manuscript. Using electron paramagnetic resonance spectroscopy to detect iron nitrosyl hemoglobin and chemiluminescent techniques to detect SNO-Hb, changes in the quaternary state of hemoglobin were found not to result in intra-molecular transfer of NO from the heme to β93 cysteine [93,94]. The lack of allosterically controlled transfer is consistent with the stability of iron nitrosyl hemoglobin upon oxygenation, which only decays with kinetics rate-limited by NO dissociation from the heme, which will be on the timeframe of tens of minutes [95]. In addition, as recognized by Stamler and colleagues [87,96], NO binds to the heme, but it must be oxidized to NO^+ for S-nitrosation. Thus, transfer from heme-NO requires an electron acceptor, and transfer from β93 cysteine requires oxidation, which could be the heme itself, but the details of these transfers are not clear. The lack of allosteric control of SNO-Hb was also demonstrated by examining its vasodilatory properties at different oxygen tensions [97], and the high oxygen affinity of SNO-Hb was suggested to reduce the likelihood that it would be deoxygenated under most physiological conditions [98]. In addition, while support for the SNO-Hb hypothesis was observed in arterial-venous gradients in SNO-Hb and iron nitrosyl hemoglobin [87,88], NO inhalation studies did not detect any arterial-venous gradient in SNO-Hb (but did observe these in both nitrite and iron nitrosyl hemoglobin) [43]. Finally, the development of a βcys93ala mutant mouse (where the β93 cysteine is replaced by an alanine) also militates against the SNO-Hb hypothesis [99]. Given the purported importance of SNO-Hb and the pathology associated with its dysfunction, one might have thought that this mutation would be lethal. However, the mice survive, and development as well as physiological function, including during exercise, were unaffected [99]. It should be noted that the red cells in the βcys93ala mice have the same amount of total nitrosothiols as wild-type, but the nitrosated species have a predominantly low molecular weight [99]. Yet, the lack of observed effects, including hypoxic vasodilation [99], despite the inability for SNO-Hb formation, argues against major aspects of the SNO-Hb hypothesis. However, other work by Stamler and colleagues showed substantial deficits in the βcys93ala mice, including cardiovascular effects and hypoxic vasodilation, which was associated with the development of pulmonary hypertension [100,101]. In another study involving multiple labs, red blood cells were shown to be able to export NO activity in a platelet, cardiac ischemia/reperfusion injury, *ex-vivo* aortic ring, and murine hypoxic vasodilation model, but this ability to transduce NO activity was not inhibited by red cells from the βcys93ala mice [102].

6   NO FERROHEME

6.1   NO FERROHEME BACKGROUND

By NO ferroheme, we mean NO bound to a ferrous (iron +2) heme. This species is known to be quite stable when bound to hemoglobin or, for example, when bound to soluble guanylate cyclase (sGC). Recall that NO binding to sGC activates the protein and constitutes a major NO signaling pathway. As early as 1985, Ignarro's group proposed nitrosyl-heme exchange as a mechanism for sGC activation, where NO ferroheme was shown to activate aposGC [103]. The Stuehr lab showed that NO ferroheme is taken up by cells relatively rapidly and can directly activate sGC [104]. The notion that nitrosyl-heme, although hydrophobic and thus requiring transport via other proteins, carries out NO signaling was recently revived in a 2017 hypothesis paper [105]. Observed arterial-venous gradients in NO ferroheme suggested the transport and signaling of these molecules [43]. NO signaling through transport of NO ferroheme could explain the export of NO activity from the red blood cell following bioactivation by nitrite [59] as well as NO signaling that occurs despite the presence of abundant oxygenated heme proteins that could inactivate NO through dioxygenation (Equation 1). Direct transfer of NO ferrous heme to activate sGC would explain how sGC can be activated when a substantial fraction of sGC exists in the aposGC form [106].

6.2 NO FERROHEME FORMATION AND CHEMISTRY

Due to its redox potential, free heme is usually in the ferric state (iron +3) and does not bind NO tightly when in this oxidized state [107]. However, ferric heme-NO can be converted to the tight NO-binding ferrous heme (NO ferroheme) by processes known as reductive nitrosylation that have been elucidated by Ford and colleagues [108]. First, NO binds the ferric heme iron, forming a species that has ferrous heme iron character bound to NO^+. This species then reacts with the hydroxyl ion to form nitrite and the reduced heme. The reduced heme can then bind NO, forming NO ferroheme. These reactions are summarized in Equations 4 and 5.

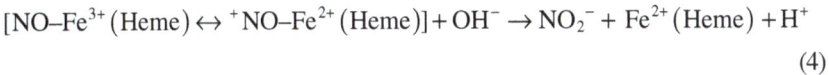

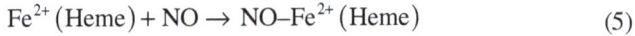

$$[NO-Fe^{3+}(Heme) \leftrightarrow {}^+NO-Fe^{2+}(Heme)] + OH^- \rightarrow NO_2^- + Fe^{2+}(Heme) + H^+ \tag{4}$$

$$Fe^{2+}(Heme) + NO \rightarrow NO-Fe^{2+}(Heme) \tag{5}$$

The kinetics of this classical reductive nitrosylation are rate-limited by the reduction of the heme, which has half-lives of minutes to tens of minutes. However, we have discovered that reductive nitrosylation is catalyzed through the involvement of a thiol such as GSH [109]. The thiol is oxidized, reducing the NO-bound ferric heme and forming a thiyl radical:

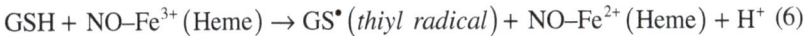

$$GSH + NO-Fe^{3+}(Heme) \rightarrow GS^\bullet (thiyl\ radical) + NO-Fe^{2+}(Heme) + H^+ \tag{6}$$

This reaction is depicted in Figure 6. The speed of this thiol-catalyzed pathway, which can occur on a millisecond-to-second time-scale, suggests its viability *in vivo*.

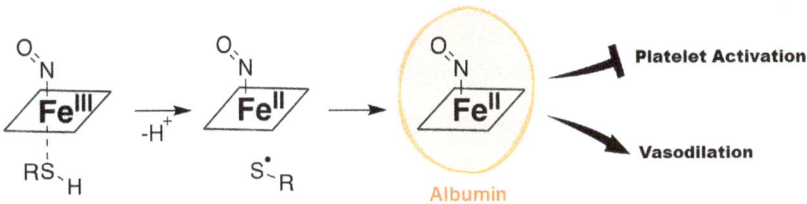

FIGURE 6 Thiol-catalyzed reductive nitrosylation. The ferric heme binds NO and binds or interacts with a thiol such as glutathione (but here shown as a generic RSH). The thiol reduces the heme nitrosyl, leaving a thiyl radical. NO ferroheme can be taken up by albumin, effect vasodilation, and inhibit platelet activation.

6.3 NO Ferroheme Signaling

As mentioned, earlier work has shown that NO ferroheme can be taken up by cells and activate sGC [103,104]. More recent work has examined NO ferroheme more thoroughly [109,110]. The thiol-catalyzed reaction was observed to proceed in the abundant heme-transporting plasma protein albumin and in membranes, as represented by red cell membrane ghosts [109]. The NO ferroheme was observed to transfer from membranes to albumin and from albumin to apo-heme proteins [109], and the NO-ferroheme myoglobin transferred NO ferroheme to aposGC and activated it [110]. NO ferroheme is stable under oxygenated conditions, including in the presence of oxyhemoglobin [109]. Studies using aortic ring bioassays demonstrated that NO ferroheme in a variety of proteins, including hemoglobin, myoglobin, and albumin, effected vasodilation that was abrogated when blocking the sGC pathway but not affected by NO scavengers, supporting cellular uptake of the NO ferroheme species and activation of sGC [110]. The NO ferroheme preparation in albumin inhibited platelet activation [109]. Finally, NO ferroheme preparations in albumin [109] or myoglobin [110] lowered blood pressure in mice [109] and rats [110]. Interestingly, the blood pressure effects of NO ferroheme albumin were potentiated by co-infusion with GSH [109].

Although establishing the physiological relevance of NO ferroheme signaling as well as therapeutic use will require substantial additional work, the robust signaling and stability of these molecules demonstrate their promise.

7 CONCLUSIONS

Heme is an essential cofactor for life that performs a multitude of functions. The fact that it performs so many important functions is due to the variety of chemical processes it can facilitate. These include ligand binding (for example, to oxygen, nitric oxide, and CO) and redox reactions such as those performed by several mitochondrial and other enzymes. Free heme, on the other hand, can be toxic. Thus, production and metabolism of heme must be tightly controlled.

In this chapter, we have described several examples of use of heme/heme proteins to develop therapeutics. Success might be considered to have been limited so far, but work is ongoing, and we expect the list of approved and practiced heme-protein–based therapeutics to increase.

ABBREVIATIONS AND DEFINTIONS

CD	cyclodextrin
cGMP	cyclic guanosine monophosphate
CO	carbon monoxide
COHb	carbon monoxide-bound hemoglobin
COX	Complex IV
DAMP	danger-associated molecular pattern

DPG	2,3-diphosphoglycerate
EMA	European Medicines Agency
FDA	Food and Drug Administration
GSH	glutathione
Hb	hemoglobin
HbO_2	oxygenated hemoglobin
HBOC	hemoglobin-based oxygen carrier
MetHb	methemoglobin
MWC	Mond-Wyman-Changeux
NEMHb	N-ethylmaleimide-bound hemoglobin
Ngb	neuroglobin
NOS	nitric oxide synthase
ROS	reactive oxygen species
sGC	soluble guanylyl (guanylate) cyclase
SNO-Hb	S-nitrosated hemoglobin
StHb	stripped hemoglobin
TL-4	toll-like receptors

REFERENCES

1. T. Shimizu, A. Lengalova, V. Martinek, M. Martinkova, *Chem. Soc. Rev.* **2019**, *48*, 5624–5657.
2. S. Janciauskiene, V. Vijayan, S. Immenschuh, *Front. Immun.* **2020**, 11.
3. K. Ishimori, Y. Watanabe, *Chem. Lett.* **2014**, *43*, 1680–1689.
4. B. Wegiel, C. J. Hauser, L. E. Otterbein, *Biol. Med.* **2015**, *89*, 651–661.
5. G. Canesin, S.M. Hejazi, K.D. Swanson, B. Wegiel, *Front. Immun.* **2020**, 11. https://www.frontiersin.org/journals/immunology/articles/10.3389/fimmu.2020.00066/full
6. L. Chen, Z. Y. Yang, H. Y. Liu, *Medicina-Lithuania* **2023**, *59*, 396. https://pubmed.ncbi.nlm.nih.gov/36837597/
7. A. S. B. Cardenas, P. P. Samuel, J. S. Olson, *Shock* **2019**, *52*, 28–40.
8. S. Faggiano, L. Ronda, S. Bruno, S. Abbruzzetti, C. Viappiani, S. Bettati, A. Mozzarelli, *Mol. Asp. Med.* **2022**, *84*, 101050. https://pubmed.ncbi.nlm.nih.gov/34776270/
9. J. Monod, J. Wyman, J. -P. Changeux, *J. Mol. Biol.* **1965**, *12*, 88–112.
10. E. R. Henry, S. Bettati, J. Hofrichter, W. A. Eaton, *Biophys. Chem.* **2002**, *98*, 149–164.
11. R. M. Winslow, *J. Intern. Med.* **2003**, *253*, 508–517.
12. L. J. Ignarro, *Nitric Oxide Biology and Pathobiology*, Academic Press, San Diego, **2000**.
13. D. H. Doherty, M. P. Doyle, S. R. Curry, R. J. Vali, T. J. Fattor, J. S. Olson, D. D. Lemon, *Nat. Biotechnol.* **1998**, *16*, 672–676.
14. J. R. Lancaster, *Natl. Acad. Sci. USA*, **1994**, *91*, 8137–8141.
15. D. B. Kim-Shapiro, A. N. Schechter, M. T. Gladwin, *Arterioscler Thromb. Vasc. Biol.* **2006**, *26*, 697–705.
16. E. Carlsen, J. H. Comroe, *J. Gen. Physiol.* **1958**, *42*, 83–107.
17. I. Azarov, K. T. Huang, S. Basu, M. T. Gladwin, N. Hogg, D. B. Kim-Shapiro, *J. Biol. Chem.* **2005**, *280*, 39024–39032. M509045200. https://pubmed.ncbi.nlm.nih.gov/16186121/

18. A. Jeffers, M. T. Gladwin, D. B. Kim-Shapiro, *Biol. Med.* **2006**, *41*, 1557–1565.
19. A. I. Alayash, *Clin. Lab. Med.* **2010**, *30*, 381–389.
20. P. W. Buehler, F. D'Agnillo, D. J. Schaer, *Trends. Mol. Med.* **2010**, *16*, 447–457.
21. A. I. Alayash, *Nat. Rev. Drug Dis.* **2004**, *3*, 152–159.
22. L. Turell, R. Radi, B. Alvarez, *Free Radic. Biol. Med.* **2013**, *65*, 244–253.
23. H. Sakai, A. Sato, P. Sobolewski, S. Takeoka, J.A. Frangos, K. Kobayashi, M. Intaglietta, E. Tsuchida, *NO and CO Binding Profiles of Hemoglobin Vesicles as Artificial Oxygen Carriers*, Elsevier Science Bv, 2008, pp. 1441–1447. https://www.sciencedirect.com/science/article/pii/S1570963908000964
24. C. Liu, W. Zhao, G. J. Christ, M. T. Gladwin, D. B. Kim-Shapiro, *Free Radic. Biol. Med.* **2013**, *65*, 1164–73.
25. H. Sakai, H. Hara, M. Yuasa, A. G. Tsai, S. Takeoka, E. Tsuchida, M. Intaglietta, *Am. J. Physiol.-Heart Circul. Physiol.* **2000**, *279*, H908–H915.
26. N. B. Charbe, F. Castillo, M. M. Tambuwala, P. Prasher, D. K. Chellappan, A. Carren, S. Satija, S. K. Singh, M. Gulati, K. Dua, J. V. Gonzalez-Aramundiz, F. C. Zacconi, *Blood Rev.* **2022**, *54*, 100927. https://www.sciencedirect.com/science/article/pii/S0268960X22000017?via%3Dihub
27. D. P. J. Pan, S. Rogers, S. Misra, G. Vulugundam, L. Gazdzinski, A. Tsui, N. Mistry, A. Said, P. Spinella, G. Hare, G. Lanza, A. Doctor, *Blood*, **2016**, *128*, 1027. https://www.sciencedirect.com/science/article/pii/S0006497119310286
28. Y. Le Meur, E. Delpy, F. Renard, T. Hauet, L. Badet, J. P. Rerolle, A. Thierry, M. Buchler, F. Zal, B. Barrou, *Artif. Organs*, **2022**, *46*, 597–605.
29. K. D. Vandegriff, M. A. Young, J. Lohman, A. Bellelli, M. Samaja, A. Malavalli, R. M. Winslow, *Br. J. Pharmacol.* **2008**, *154*, 1649–1661.
30. S. J. Wolf, E. J. Lavonas, E. P. Sloan, A. S. Jagoda, W. W. Decker, D. B. Diercks, J. A. Edlow, F. M. Fesmire, S. A. Godwin, S. A. Hahn, J. M. Howell, J. S. Huff, T. W. Lukens, D. L. Mason, M. Moon, A. M. Napoli, D. Nazarian, J. Richmann, S. M. Silvers, M. E. W. Thiessen, R. L. Wears, C. D. Hobgood, D. C. Seaberg, R. R. Whitson, P. *Ann. Emerg. Med.* **2008**, *51*, 138–152.
31. J. J. Rose, L. Wang, Q. Z. Xu, C. F. McTiernan, S. Shiva, J. Tejero, M. T. Gladwin, *Am. J. Respir. Crit. Care Med.* **2017**, *195*, 596–606.
32. I. Azarov, L. Wang, J. J. Rose, Q. Xu, X. N. Huang, A. Belanger, Y. Wang, L. Guo, C. Liu, K. B. Ucer, C. F. McTiernan, C. P. O'Donnell, S. Shiva, J. Tejero, D. B. Kim-Shapiro, M. T. Gladwin, *Sci. Transl. Med.* **2016**, *8*, 368ra173.
33. C. A. Piantadosi, in, *Carbon Monoxide*, Ed.: D. G. Penney, CRC-Taylor and Francis Press, New York, **1996**.https://www.taylorfrancis.com/chapters/edit/10.1201/9780429260674-8/toxicity-carbon-monoxide-hemoglobin-vs-histo-toxic-mechanisms-claude-piantadosi?context=ubx&refId=9cf96575-a0c0-4cd7-a499-b73243cf6e7d
34. Q. Mao, X. Zhao, A. Kiriyama, H. Kitagashi, *Proc. Natl. Acad. Sci. USA*, **2023**, *120*, e2209924120.
35. D. K. Quinn, M. M. Shunda, P. C. Laura, G. N. Duncan, C. Cusin, C. J. Hopwood, T. A. Stern, *Prim. Care Comp. J. Clin. Psychiatry*, **2009**, *11*, 74–79.
36. E. P. Sloan, D. G. Murphy, R. Hart, M. A. Cooper, T. Turnbull, R. S. Barreca, B. Ellerson, *Ann. Emer. Med.* **1989**, *18*, 629–634.
37. J. J. Rose, K. A. Bocian, Q. Z. Xu, L. Wang, A. W. DeMartino, X. K. Chen, C. G. Corey, D. A. Guimaraes, I. Azarov, X. Y. N. Huang, Q. Tong, L. P. Guo, M. Nouraie, C. F. McTiernan, C. P. O'Donnell, J. Tejero, S. Shiva, M. T. Gladwin, *J. Biol. Chem.* **2020**, *295*, 6357–6371.

38. Q. Z. Xu, J. J. Rose, X. K. Chen, L. Wang, A. W. DeMartino, M. R. Dent, S. Tiwari, K. Bocian, X. N. Huang, Q. Tong, C. F. McTiernan, L. P. Guo, E. Alipour, T. C. Jones, K. B. Ucer, D. B. Kim-Shapiro, J. Tejero, M. T. Gladwin, *Jci. Insight*, **2022**, 7.
39. D. G. Droege, T. C. Johnstone, *Chem. Commun.* **2022**, *58*, 2722–2725.
40. H. Kitagishi, S. Minegishi, A. Yumura, S. Negi, S. Taketani, Y. Amagase, Y. Mizukawa, T. Urushidani, Y. Sugiura, K. Kano, *J. Am. Chem. Soc.* **2016**, *138*, 5417–5425.
41. Q. Y. Mao, A. T. Kawaguchi, S. Mizobata, R. Motterlini, R. Foresti, H. Kitagishi, *Commun. Biol.* **2021**, *4*. https://www.nature.com/articles/s42003-021-01880-1
42. H. Kitagishi, S. Negi, A. Kiriyama, A. Honbo, Y. Sugiura, A. T. Kawaguchi, K. Kano, *Angew. Chem. Int. Ed.* **2010**, *49*, 1312–1315.
43. M. T. Gladwin, F. P. Ognibene, L. K. Pannell, J. S. Nichols, M. E. Pease-Fye, J. H. Shelhamer, A. N. Schechter, *Proc. Natl. Acad. Sci. USA.* **2000**, *97*, 9943–9948.
44. M. T. Gladwin, J. H. Shelhamer, A. N. Schechter, M. E. Pease-Fye, M. A. Waclawiw, J. A. Panza, F. P. Ognibene, R. O. Cannon, *Circulation* **2000**, *102*, 172–173.
45. T. Lauer, M. Preik, T. Rassaf, B. E. Strauer, A. Deussen, M. Feelisch, M. Kelm, *Natl. Acad. Sci. USA*, **2001**, *98*, 12814–12819.
46. K. Cosby, K. S. Partovi, J. H. Crawford, R. P. Patel, C. D. Reiter, S. Martyr, B. K. Yang, M. A. Waclawiw, G. Zalos, X. Xu, K. T. Huang, H. Shields, D. B. Kim-Shapiro, A. N. Schechter, R. O. Cannon, 3rd, M. T. Gladwin, *Nat. Med.* **2003**, *9*, 1498–1505.
47. A. Dejam, C. J. Hunter, C. Tremonti, R. M. Pluta, Y. Y. Hon, G. Grimes, K. Partovi, M. M. Pelletier, E. H. Oldfield, R. O. Cannon, III, A. N. Schechter, M. T. Gladwin, *Circulation*, **2007**, 116, 1821–1831.
48. J. Brooks, *Proc. Royal Soc. London - Series B, Biol. Sci.* **1937**, *123*, 368–382.
49. M. P. Doyle, R. A. Pickering, T. M. Deweert, J. W. Hoekstra, D. Pater, *J. Biol. Chem.* **1981**, *256*, 12393–12398.
50. J. L. Zweier, P. H. Wang, A. Samouilov, P. Kuppusamy, *Nat. Med.* **1995**, *1*, 804–809.
51. A. Modin, H. Bjorne, M. Herulf, K. Alving, E. Weitzberg, J. O. N. Lundberg, *Acta Physiol. Scand.* 2001 *171*, 9–16.
52. Z. Huang, S. Shiva, D. B. Kim-Shapiro, R. P. Patel, L. A. Ringwood, C. E. Irby, K. T. Huang, C. Ho, N. Hogg, A. N. Schechter, M. T. Gladwin, *J. Clin. Invest.* **2005**, *115*, 2099–2107.
53. K. T. Huang, A. Keszler, N. Patel, R. P. Patel, M. T. Gladwin, D. B. Kim-Shapiro, N. Hogg, *J. Biol. Chem.* **2005**, *280*, 31126–31131.
54. M. T. Gladwin, J. H. Crawford, R. P. Patel, *Free Radic. Biol. Med.* **2004**, *36*, 707–717.
55. S. Basu, R. Grubina, J. Huang, J. Conradie, Z. Huang, A. Jeffers, A. Jiang, X. He, I. Azarov, R. Seibert, A. Mehta, R. Patel, S. B. King, N. Hogg, A. Ghosh, M. T. Gladwin, D. B. Kim-Shapiro, *Nat. Chem. Biol.* **2007**, *3*, 785–94.
56. E. Nagababu, S. Ramasamy, J. M. Rifkind, *Biochem.-US*, **2007**, *46*, 11650–11659.
57. M. Angelo, D. J. Singel, J. S. Stamler, *Natl. Acad. Sci. USA*, **2006**, *103*, 8366–8371.
58. N. Wajih, X. Liu, P. Shetty, S. Basu, H. Wu, N. Hogg, R. P. Patel, C. M. Furdui, D. B. Kim-Shapiro, *Redox. Biol.* **2016**, *8*, 415–21.
59. N. Wajih, S. Basu, K. B. Ucer, F. Rigal, A. Shakya, E. Rahbar, V. Vachharajani, M. Guthold, M. T. Gladwin, L. M. Smith, D. B. Kim-Shapiro, *Redox. Biol.* **2019**, *20*, 442–450.
60. J. H. Crawford, T. S. Isbell, Z. Huang, S. Shiva, B. K. Chacko, A. N. Schechter, V. M. Darley-Usmar, J. D. Kerby, J. D. Lang Jr, D. Kraus, C. Ho, M. T. Gladwin, R. P. Patel, *Blood*, **2006**, *15*, 566–574.

61. S. Shiva, T. Rassaf, R. P. Patel, M. T. Gladwin, *Res.* **2011**, *89*, 566–573.
62. S. Srihirun, T. Sriwantana, S. Unchern, D. Kittikool, E. Noulsri, K. Pattanapanyasat, S. Fucharoen, B. Piknova, A. N. Schechter, N. Sibmooh *PLoS One*, **2012**, *7*, e30380.
63. R. M. Pluta, E. H. Oldfield, K. D. Bakhtian, A. R. Fathi, R. K. Smith, H. L. DeVroom, M. Nahavandi, S. Woo, W. D. Figg, R. R. Lonser, *PLoS One* **2011**, *6*, e14504.
64. R. M. Pluta, A. Dejam, G. Grimes, M. T. Gladwin, E. H. Oldfield, *J. Am. Med. Assoc.-JAMA*, **2005**, *293*, 1477–1484.
65. M. R. Duranski, J. J. M. Greer, A. Dejam, S. Jaganmohan, N. Hogg, W. Langston, R. P. Patel, S. F. Yet, X. D. Wang, C.G. Kevil, M. T. Gladwin, D. J. Lefer, *J. Clin. Invest.* **2005**, *115*, 1232–1240.
66. T. E. Ingram, A. G. Fraser, R. A. Bleasdale, E. A. Ellins, A. D. Margulescu, J. P. Halcox, P. E. James, *J. Am. Coll. Cardiol.* **2013**, *61*, 2534–2541.
67. A. K. Mack, V. R. McGowan, C. K. Tremonti, D. Ackah, C. Barnett, R. F. Machado, M. T. Gladwin, G. J. Kato, *Brit. J. Haematol.* **2008**, *142*, 971–978.
68. N. Wajih, S. Basu, A. Jailwala, H. W. Kim, D. Ostrowski, A. Perlegas, C. A. Bolden, N. L. Buechler, M. T. Gladwin, D. L. Caudell, E. Rahbar, M. A. Alexander-Miller, V. Vachharajani, D. B. Kim-Shapiro, *Redox. Biol.* **2017**, *12*, 1026–1039.
69. B. A. Borlaug, V. Melenovsky, K. E. Koepp, *Res.* **2016**, *119*, 880–886.
70. K. S. Hughan, A. Levine, N. Helbling, S. Anthony, J. P. DeLany, M. Stefanovic-Racic, B. H. Goodpaster, M. T. Gladwin, *Hypertension*, **2020**, *76*, 866–874.
71. J. O. Lundberg, E. Weitzberg, M. T. Gladwin, *Nat. Rev. Drug. Discov.* **2008**, *7*, 156–67.
72. T. D. Presley, A. R. Morgan, E. Bechtold, W. Clodfelter, R. W. Dove, J. M. Jennings, R. A. Kraft, S. B. King, P. J. Laurienti, W. J. Rejeski, J. H. Burdette, D. B. Kim-Shapiro, G. D. Miller, *Nitric Oxide* **2011**, *24*, 34–42.
73. M. Petrie, W.J. Rejeski, S. Basu, P. J. Laurienti, A. P. Marsh, J. L. Norris, D. B. Kim-Shapiro, J. H. Burdette, *J. Geront. A*, **2017**, *72*, 1284–1289.
74. M. Berry, N. W. Justus, J. I. Hauser, A. H. Case, C. C. H. S. Basu, Z. Rogers, M. T. Lewis, G. D. Miller, *Nitric Oxide* **2014**, doi: 10.1016/j.niox.2014.10.007.
75. J. Eggebeen, D. B. Kim-Shapiro, M. Haykowsky, T. M. Morgan, S. Basu, P. Brubaker, J. Rejeski, D. W. Kitzman, *JACC Heart Fail.* **2016**, *4*, 428–37.
76. P. Zamani, D. Rawat, P. Shiva-Kumar, S. Geraci, R. Bhuva, P. Konda, P. T. Doulias, H. Ischiropoulos, R. R. Townsend, K. B. Margulies, T. P. Cappola, D. C. Poole, J. A. Chirinos, *Circulation* **2015**, *131*, 371–U1184.
77. S. Velmurugan, V. Kapil, S. M. Ghosh, S. Davies, A. McKnight, Z. Aboud, R. S. Khambata, A. J. Webb, A. Poole, A. Ahluwalia, *Biol. Med.* **2013**, *65*, 1521–1532.
78. C. Rammos, U. B. Hendgen-Cotta, J. Sobierajski, A. Bernard, M. Kelm, T. Rassaf, *J. Am. Coll. Cardiol.* **2014**, *63*, 1584–1585.
79. A. A. Kenjale, K. L. Ham, T. Stabler, J. L. Robbins, J. L. Johnson, M. VanBruggen, G. Privette, E. Yim, W. E. Kraus, J. D. Allen, *J. Appl. Physiol.* **2011**, *110*, 1582–1591.
80. M. Woessner, M. D. VanBruggen, C. F. Pieper, R. Sloane, W. E. Kraus, A. J. Gow, J. D. Allen, *Circ. Res.* **2018**, *123*, 654–659.
81. J. M. Bock, D. P. Treichler, S. L. Norton, K. Ueda, W. E. Hughes, D. P. Casey, *Nitric. Oxide-Biol. Ch.* **2018**, *80*, 45–51.
82. V. Kapil, R. S. Khambata, A. Robertson, M. J. Caulfield, A. Ahluwalia, *Hypertension* **2015**, *65*, 320–U174.
83. O. Esen, N. Dobbin, M. J. Callaghan, *J. Am. Nut. Assoc.* **2023**, *42*, 327–338.
84. C. M. Meirelles, K. F. Spaolonse, *Rbne-Revista Brasileira De Nutricao Esportiva*, **2023**, *17*, 11–21.

85. S. J. Bailey, P. Winyard, A. Vanhatalo, J. R. Blackwell, F. J. DiMenna, D. P. Wilkerson, J. Tarr, N. Benjamin, A. M. Jones, *J. Appl. Physiol.* **2009**, *107*, 1144–1155.
86. F. J. Larsen, E. Weitzberg, J. O. Lundberg, B. Ekblom, *Biol. Med.* **2010**, *48*, 342–347.
87. L. Jia, C. Bonaventura, J. Bonaventura, J. S. Stamler, *Nature* **1996**, *380*, 221–226.
88. T. J. McMahon, R. E. Moon, B. P. Luschinger, M. S. Carraway, A. E. Stone, B. W. Stolp, A. J. Gow, J. R. Pawloski, P. Watke, D. J. Singel, C. A. Piantadosi, J. S. Stamler, *Nat. Med.* **2002**, *8*, 711–717.
89. J. R. Pawloski, D. T. Hess, J. S. Stamler, *Natl. Acad. Sci. USA* **2005**, *102*, 2531–2536.
90. T. J. McMahon, G. S. Ahearn, M. P. Moya, A. J. Gow, Y.- C. T. Huang, B. P. Luchsinger, R. Nudelman, Y. Yan, A. D. Krichman, T. M. Bashore, R. M. Califf, D. J. Singel, C. A. Piantadosi, V. F. Tapson, J. S. Stamler, *Natl. Acad. Sci. USA* **2005**, *102*, 14801–14806.
91. J. D. Reynolds, G. S. Ahearn, M. Angelo, J. Zhang, F. Cobb, J. S. Stamler, *Natl. Acad. Sci. USA* **2007**, *104*, 17058–17062.
92. J. D. Reynolds, K. M. Bennett, A. J. Cina, D. L. Diesen, M. B. Henderson, F. Matto, A. Plante, R. A. Williamson, K. Zandinejad, I. T. Demchenko, D. T. Hess, C. A. Piantadosi, J. S. Stamler, *. Natl. Acad. Sci. USA* **2013**, *110*, 11529–11534.
93. X. L. Xu, M. Cho, N. Y. Spencer, N. Patel, Z. Huang, H. Shields, S. B. King, M. T. Gladwin, N. Hogg, D. B. Kim-Shapiro, *Proc.* Natl. Acad. Sci. USA **2003**, *100*, 11303–11308.
94. K. T. Huang, I. Azarov, S. Basu, J. Huang, D. B. Kim-Shapiro, *Blood* **2006**, *107*, 2602–2604.
95. F. Azizi, J. E. Kielbasa, A. M. Adeyiga, R. D. Maree, M. Frazier, M. Yakubu, H. Shields, S. B. King, D. B. Kim-Shapiro, *Biol. Med.* **2005**, *39*, 145–151.
96. B. P. Luchsinger, E. N. Rich, A. J. Gow, E. M. Williams, J. S. Stamler, D. J. Singel, *Proc.* Natl. Acad. Sci. USA **2003**, *100*, 461–466.
97. J. H. Crawford, C. R. White, R. P. Patel, *Blood* **2003**, *101*, 4408–4415.
98. R. P. Patel, N. Hogg, N. Y. Spencer, B. Kalyanaraman, S. Matalon, V. M. Darley-Usmar, *J. Biol. Chem.* **1999**, *274*, 15487–15492.
99. T. S. Isbell, C. W. Sun, L. C. Wu, X. J. Teng, D. A. Vitturi, B. G. Branch, C. G. Kevil, N. Peng, J. M. Wyss, N. Ambalavanan, L. Schwiebert, J. X. Ren, K. M. Pawlik, M. B. Renfrow, R. P. Patel, T. M. Townes, *Nat. Med.* **2008**, *14*, 773–777.
100. R. L. Zhang, A. Hausladen, Z. X. Qian, X. D. Liao, R. T. Premont, J. S. Stamler, *Jci. Insight.* **2022**, *7*. https://insight.jci.org/articles/view/155234
101. R. T. Premont, J. S. Stamler, *Physiology* **2020**, *35*, 234–243.
102. C. W. Sun, J. N. Yang, A. L. Kleschyov, Z. B. Zhuge, M. Carlstrom, J. Pernow, N. Wajih, T. S. Isbell, J. Y. Oh, P. Cabrales, A. G. Tsai, T. Townes, D. B. Kim-Shapiro, R. P. Patel, J. O. Lundberg, *Circulation* **2019**, *139*, 2654–2663.
103. L. J. Ignarro, J. B. Adams, P. M. Horwitz, K. S. Wood, *J. Biol. Chem.* **1986**, *261*, 4997–5002.
104. E. A. Sweeny, A. P. Hunt, A. E. Batka, S. Schlanger, N. Lehnert, D. J. Stuehr, *Biol. Med.* **2021**, *172*, 252–263.
105. A. L. Kleschyov, *Biol. Med.* **2017**, *112*, 544–552.
106. D. J. Stuehr, S. Misra, Y. Dai, A. Ghosh, *J. Biol. Chem.* **2021**, *296*.
107. C. E. Cooper, *Biochim. Biophys. Acta-Bioenerg.* **1999**, *1411*, 290–309.
108. M. Hoshino, M. Maeda, R. Konishi, H. Seki, P. C. Ford, *J. Am. Chem. Soc.* **1996**, *118*, 5702–5707.
109. A. DeMartino, L. Poudel, M. Dent, X. Chen, Q. Xu, B. Gladwin, J. Tejero, S. Basu, E. Alipour, Y. Jiang, J. Rose, M. Gladwin, D. Kim-Shapiro, *Res. Sq.* **2023**. https://pubmed.ncbi.nlm.nih.gov/36711928

110. A. Kleschyov, Z. Zhuge, T. Schiffer, D. Guimarães, G. Zhang, M. Montenegro, A. Tesse, E. Weitzberg, M. Carlström, J. Lundberg, *Res. Sq.* **2023**. https://www.researchsquare.com/article/rs-2529377/v1
111. L. S. Ma, L. Hu, X. Y. Feng, S. L. Wang, *Aging Dis.* **2018**, *9*, 938–945.
112. M. M. Grant, D. Jonsson, *J. Clin. Med.* **2019**, *8*. https://www.mdpi.com/2077-0383/8/8/1110

6 Metal-Containing and Metal-Associated Dietary Nutrients

Rebeca L. Fernandez[#]

Department of Chemistry
University of California, Davis
Davis, California 95616, USA

Vanessa J. Lee[#]

Department of Chemistry
University of California, Davis
Davis, California 95616, USA

Marie C. Heffern[*]

Department of Chemistry
University of California, Davis
Davis, California 95616, USA
mcheffern@ucdavis.edu

CONTENTS

[#] These authors contributed equally.
[*] Corresponding author.

DOI: 10.1201/9781003361756-6

ABSTRACT

Metal ions are key components for proper biological function, playing key roles as structural and catalytic cofactors in biomolecules while also impacting biological redox balance. As metals can neither be created nor destroyed, humans must acquire them from the diet, and their chemistry and bioavailability must be properly regulated within the body to perform their functions. This chapter provides an overview of our understanding of metals as micronutrients as well as their interaction with other classes of micronutrients, vitamins, and other natural products in nutrition. While many questions remain unanswered regarding the molecular mechanisms underpinning the relationships between metals and nutritional components, this overview points to open areas within this topic for which emerging analytical and chemical biology tools might be applied.

KEYWORDS

Micronutrient; Mineral; Vitamin; Metal Regulation; Nutrition; Iron; Cobalt; Zinc

1   INTRODUCTION

Human life requires us to obtain nutrients through food. These nutrients can be classified into two categories: macronutrients, which make up the bulk of our food, and micronutrients. Macronutrients, like proteins, carbohydrates, and lipids, are broken down by our bodies into usable energy sources [1]. In contrast, micronutrients are required in much smaller amounts than macronutrients and yet still play vital roles in maintaining homeostatic processes. The term micronutrients comprises vitamins and minerals; vitamins are produced by plants and animals and are metabolized in the human body, whereas minerals are inorganic in nature and cannot be broken down [2]. Although required in smaller amounts than macronutrients, their lower concentrations make their tight balance critical, with slight changes in micronutrient levels resulting in dyshomeostasis and disease. Their trace levels have complicated their study, but increasingly analytical and chemical biology methods are starting to reveal new roles for micronutrients, both as independent components as well as their interactions with one another and with macronutrients. This rise in knowledge has especially benefited our understanding of mineral components with the development of sophisticated new tools for quantitation, speciation, and live-cell monitoring of metal ions in cells. This chapter provides a general overview of the current understanding of minerals as they relate to nutrition, along with some highlighted examples of metal-associated micronutrients and the effects that their dysregulation can cause on the human body. We note that many of the associations are largely observational, with mechanistic understanding remaining in its infancy, but delineating these known relationships offers a starting point for directions that the new emerging tools can illuminate.

2   MINERAL MICRONUTRIENTS

In a nutritional context, minerals encompass elements from the periodic table that are essential for life. Mineral micronutrients include main-group elements (e.g., boron, silicon, iodine), alkaline earth metals (e.g., magnesium, calcium), alkali metals (e.g., sodium, potassium), and d-block metals (e.g., copper, iron, cobalt, zinc, manganese, nickel). Essential minerals can be classified into two groups: major minerals and trace minerals. The major minerals, which are used and stored in large quantities in the body, constitute calcium, chloride, magnesium, phosphorus, potassium, sodium, and sulfur. Trace minerals, which are also vital just in smaller concentrations, include chromium, copper, fluoride, iodine, iron, manganese, molybdenum, selenium, and zinc.

Unlike their vitamin counterparts, mineral micronutrients cannot be biochemically synthesized in the body [1]. These elements are found in a variety of foods, spanning dairy products, meats, fruits, and vegetables. Minerals that are not manufactured by the organisms we eat absorb micronutrients from the rocks, soil, and water that help plants grow, and in turn, animals intake these elements upon plant consumption (Figure 1). While fresh foods are one source of dietary minerals, some processed foods, like breakfast cereal, may be fortified with minerals. Mineral supplements in the form of pills, powders, and chewables

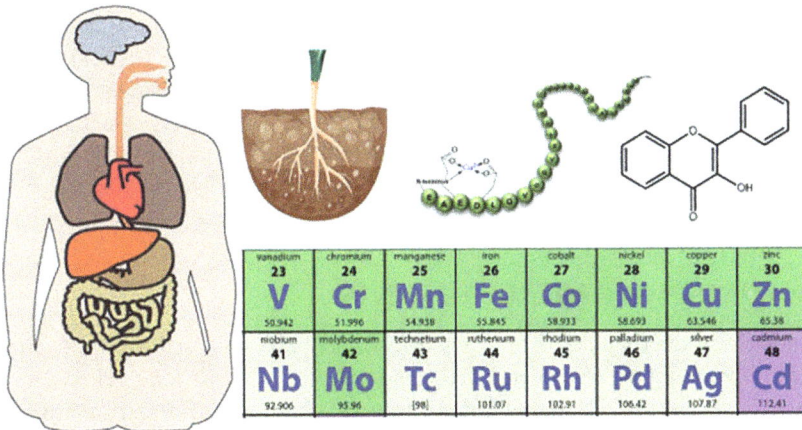

FIGURE 1   Nutritional minerals encompass trace elements like transition metals and, importantly, are obtained from diet consumption. Plants, in turn, absorb minerals from their environment.

are common, although similar to vitamins, the absorption of these micronutrients is less understood and can be less effective than bioavailable sources.

3   THE MAIN-GROUP MINERALS

While all mineral micronutrients are considered trace in terms of their quantities, the main-group minerals are found in higher concentrations relative to their d-block counterparts. Calcium is one of the most commonly touted mineral micronutrients that is associated with bone health [1]. Indeed, bones and teeth store this element for its use through blood transport elsewhere in the body. Calcium participates in the named calcium channels that regulate cell signaling [3]. Notably, proper calcium channel maintenance is required for cardiovascular function and muscle activity. The most well-known disease linked to calcium deficiency is osteoporosis, which is characterized by the loss of bone mass [4]. While genetic factors do play a role in osteoporosis, calcium intake can mitigate the risk of disease onset. We consume calcium in dairy products, leafy greens, legumes, and nuts. Similar to calcium, potassium channels traffic potassium ions and induce electrochemical gradients to control biochemical processes like cell signaling [5]. Potassium is famously found in bananas, though it is also present in other fruits such as oranges and avocados [1]. Due to the functions of potassium channels, potassium deficiency is linked to muscle cramps and cardiovascular disease relating to improperly regulated electrochemical gradients.

Another s-block element cation, sodium, has ion channels that are responsible for forming action potentials in excitable cells [6]. Participating in neuronal and cardiovascular pathways, sodium is required for the maintenance of human life. Sodium is sufficiently obtained through diet, perhaps in excess with the addition of table salt and sodium chloride. Though rare, sodium deficiency (hyponatremia) can occur in instances of excessive sweating, diarrhea, vomiting, and kidney disease [7]. Hyponatremia presents as symptoms of muscle weakness, cramps, and nausea. The counterion to sodium in table salt, chloride, is an anionic micronutrient. Channels that traffic chloride across cell membranes are found in tracheal, airway, and nasal epithelial cells [8]. Chloride also plays a key role in managing cell volume through hydration mechanisms, and its dysregulation is linked to cystic fibrosis [9]. Fluoride, an anion famously linked to dental health, is required for the mineralization of teeth and bones [10]. Fluoride is often obtained through drinking water and can be supplemented to prevent fluoride deficiency–associated tooth decay.

4   THE D-BLOCK MICRONUTRIENTS

Main-group micronutrients are touted for their beneficial health effects, while their d-block metal equivalents are classically regarded as toxic. However, as analytical methods for studying these minerals have emerged and improved, a growing body of information is revealing the nuances of their essentiality, including the detrimental effects associated with their dietary deficiencies. While redox-active metal micronutrients may exhibit toxic effects when dysregulated, they play many integral roles in maintaining proper function of human biology.

Transition metals like copper, chromium, iron, manganese, and zinc are essential for living beings as they play crucial roles in various metabolic functions, enzymatic activities, hormonal regulation, and protein transport. Other elements like arsenic, cadmium, and lead are non-essential, and low levels can have deleterious effects on plants, animals, and humans. Metal micronutrients, including copper, iron, and zinc, are minerals that are unable to be broken down in the body [11]. They function as structural cofactors, serve as redox centers, and participate in intra- and extracellular signaling. In this section, we describe the trace minerals, iron, zinc, and cobalt (in vitamin B_{12}), which are the most well-studied in terms of the effects of their deficiencies, but also describe the essentiality of copper from the lens of the metabolic impacts of its dysregulation.

4.1 IRON

The most widely recognized d-block metal micronutrient is likely iron. Iron binds to hemoglobin and is essential for respiration and oxygen transport within the body [12]. Iron is also involved in DNA synthesis and participates in redox reactions in both cells and the blood. When dysregulation occurs in iron metabolism, redox-active iron ions can participate in Fenton chemistry, resulting in damaging oxidative stress. Iron is consumed through diet, often in meat, legumes, fruits, and vegetables [13]. When an insufficient amount of iron is consumed, the body may experience iron deficiency, in which there is no stored iron accessible [14]. Iron deficiency often leads to anemia, which affects cognitive function and the immune system. Anemia can be treated with an increase in iron consumption through diet and supplements [13]. While iron deficiency can cause anemia and related health concerns, iron overload is often linked to metabolic disease states, including type 2 diabetes and non-alcoholic fatty liver disease (NAFLD) [15]. The unknown mechanisms of iron metabolism under pathological conditions continue to be investigated by labs around the world.

4.2 ZINC

Unlike iron, zinc is not redox-active due to its full d-orbital electron count. Zinc is obtained through diet and is found in high levels in oysters, red meat, and poultry. Zinc participates in human biology as a metal cofactor and transcriptional regulator, affecting functions ranging from immune response to bone growth [11]. Zinc metalloenzymes continue to be discovered, and the most widely recognized zinc-containing proteins are called zinc finger proteins [16]. Zinc finger proteins were first discovered as nuclear transcriptional factors and can bind DNA. These transcription factors regulate processes including stem cell maintenance, cell proliferation, gluconeogenesis, and adipogenesis. Zinc is also employed in insulin storage, as this metal stabilizes a trimer of insulin dimers [17,18]. Thus, it is no surprise that zinc dysregulation is associated with metabolic diseases, most notably diabetes. Zinc deficiency is linked to high glucose levels, though the mechanisms of zinc regulation under diabetic states remain poorly characterized.

4.3   COBALAMIN (VITAMIN B$_{12}$)

While most metals are consumed in mineral form, the notable exception is cobalt, which is consumed in the form of vitamin B$_{12}$ (Figure 2) [19]. Organisms in all life domains require B$_{12}$, although fungi, plants, and animals are unable to synthesize this micronutrient. Vitamin B$_{12}$, or cobalamin, serves as a cofactor for the two enzymes: methionine synthase and methylmalonyl-CoA mutase. In these enzymes, which participate in methylation processes, the cofactor consists of a hexacoordinate cobalt ion equatorially bound by four nitrogens in the corrin macrocycle and a methyl group in the upper axial position. This methyl group is transferred during enzymatic reactions important to DNA synthesis and nerve maintenance [20]. Like with its mineral counterparts, dysregulation of vitamin B$_{12}$ is related to health issues including pernicious anemia and Chron's disease. In the blood, the majority of cobalamin is bound by two proteins: 80% to haptocorrin and 20% to transcobalamin [21]. Cobalamin bound to HC (holoHC) is not considered bioavailable due to the lack of a receptor on the cell surface; cobalamin bound to transcobalamin can be internalized and is considered the bioactive form of cobalamin [22]. Vitamin B$_{12}$ deficiency is linked to disease states including pernicious anemia and neurological diseases such as Parkinson's and Alzheimer's, but the underlying mechanisms of these pathologies remain elusive. Despite its importance, few methods are available for tracking cobalamin *in vivo*, and state-of-the-art clinical assays require lengthy times and lack important information about the bioavailability of B$_{12}$ in the body, thereby limiting our understanding of B$_{12}$ regulation and status [23].

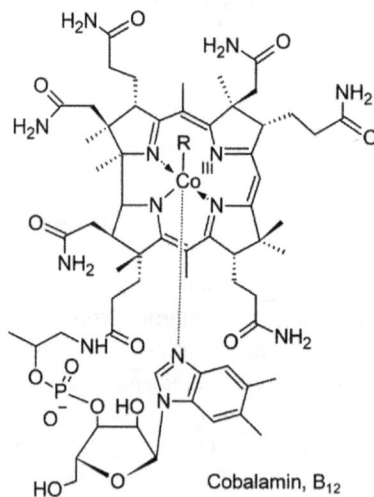

Cobalamin, B$_{12}$

FIGURE 2   Chemical structure of Co^{III} cobalamins. The biologically available form of cobalamin, vitamin B$_{12}$, is cyanocobalamin, in which the upper axial ligand, denoted R, is a cyanide moiety.

4.4 MICRONUTRIENT IMBALANCE IN DISEASE: THE EXAMPLE OF COPPER DYSREGULATION IN METABOLIC DISEASE STATES

Copper, like the aforementioned d-block metals, serves as a cofactor for a host of enzymes in the body [24]. Roles as static cofactors in oxygenases, hydrolases, and transferases take advantage of the redox-active nature of copper. Notably, copper serves as a cofactor to cytochrome c oxidase, which is involved in respiration through electron transfer [25]. Copper is tightly regulated because, like iron, aberrant copper species can produce reactive oxygen species via Fenton-like chemistry and, in turn, cause oxidative stress. Copper is obtained from consumption of foods like oysters, spinach, and dark chocolate and is trafficked through the body by chaperones in the blood and cytosol and transmembrane transporters [26]. While tightly bound copper is required for the proper function of cuproenzymes, whether labile or more loosely bound, copper is importantly modulated in metabolic disease states [27].

While necessary to maintain proper function, copper can exhibit toxic effects if it is not tightly regulated. As such, copper dysregulation is related to a host of disease states, including metabolic disorders and cancer. This element is increasingly being recognized for its role in signaling and functions derived from labile copper pools [28]. The two most studied genetic diseases in which metal transport is affected include Menkes' and Wilson's diseases, where patients have mutations in copper exporters ATP7A and ATP7B, respectively [29,30]. Patients with Menkes' disease have low copper levels in their serum, liver, and brain, which presents symptoms including hypopigmented hair, respiratory failure, and vascular complications [31]. Conversely, patients with Wilson's disease have high serum copper levels and can experience steatosis or cirrhosis without timely treatment [32]. Chronic metabolic diseases like NAFLD and type 2 diabetes do not have direct relationships to metal metabolism, but patients often exhibit altered clinical metal levels [18,33].

NAFLD incidences are fast rising across the world, with the disease characterized by fat deposits within the liver [34]. If allowed to progress without intervention, NAFLD can lead to irreversible liver damage from non-alcoholic steatohepatitis, cirrhosis, and hepatocellular carcinoma. Patients with NAFLD clinically present with lower serum copper levels [33]. *In vivo* studies demonstrate that copper deficiency is linked to changes in metabolism and mitochondrial function [35]. As such, there is a need to understand the underlying causal relationships between copper dysregulation and NAFLD in order to develop better treatment plans. The Heffern lab investigated the effects of fatty acids on copper status in the liver by treating hepatic cells with a saturated fatty acid (palmitic acid) [36]. Changes in copper trafficking caused by these stimulations ultimately led to copper deficiency in the cell. A detailed understanding of the biological mechanisms and a precise, chemical understanding of the factors at play can be harnessed to develop therapeutics that target involved proteins or improperly localized copper.

Copper trafficking molecules are currently employed for treatment of diseases, including Wilson's and Menkes' diseases [37]. Specifically, copper chelators are used, which bind copper for excretion from the body, thereby preventing copper overload. Chelators such as tetrathiomolybdate, trientine, and D-penicillamine are clinically prescribed with promising results. Further investigation is warranted to discover copper trafficking molecules that reorganize copper within the body rather than excrete the ions, given that copper mislocalization is often associated with disease [30]. Toward this end, copper-binding molecules inspired by plant natural products are being investigated for their potential nutraceutical effects [38–40], which are further detailed in Section 6.

5   VITAMINS AND POSSIBLE LINKS TO MINERAL AVAILABILITY

The bioavailability of minerals and vitamins has been demonstrated to affect one another, but by and large, their interactions are observational, with a heavy focus on iron and zinc availability and with molecular connections yet to be determined. Vitamins are obtained through our food intake and perform a wide range of biological activities, including serving as cofactors, regulating cell growth, and imparting antioxidant activity. Their diverse roles, in conjunction with the lack of tools to study their biological levels, contribute to the challenge of dissecting cause from effect with respect to how their supplementation and status may affect mineral availability. Thus, many of the studies associating minerals with vitamins focus on either the effects of their supplementation or the concomitance of their deficiencies [2]. This section provides an overview of the vitamins and summarizes the limited knowledge regarding interactions with the common minerals.

5.1   VITAMIN A AND POSSIBLE LINKS TO IRON AND ZINC

The vitamin A class includes retinoids and carotenoids, which play key roles in physiological processes such as vision, reproduction, embryonic growth and development, immune competence, cell differentiation, cell proliferation and apoptosis, maintenance of epithelial tissue, and brain function [2]. Retinoids are derivatives of naturally occurring vitamin A, which exists as retinol or retinyl esters (Figure 3a). Retinoids contain four isoprenoid units, and vitamin A is the all-*trans* parent molecule [1]. Vitamin A is a fat-soluble vitamin that is found in milk, eggs, and beef liver [41]. Aside from the role of this micronutrient subclass in vision, much of the affected cellular processes arise from vitamin A and its analogs binding to receptors and retinoid metabolizing enzymes [42].

The remainder of the vitamin A class consists of carotenoids, which are composed of eight isoprenoid units with an inversion center and derive from acyclic $C_{40}H_{56}$ (Figure 3b). Carotenoids are mainly found in photosynthetic plants and algae, as opposed to their animal-derived retinol counterparts [43]. The class of vitamin A molecules is required for the maintenance of many tissues in the body, but their most well-known function is in the eye [44]. In the retina, rhodopsin, a G-protein–coupled receptor, binds vitamin A in the form of 11-*cis*-retinal.

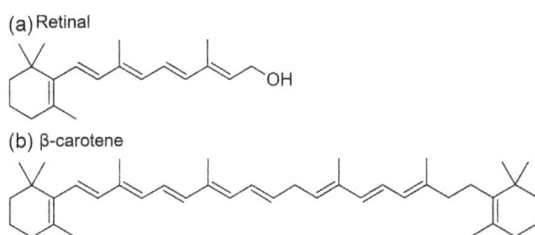

FIGURE 3 Vitamin A molecules are derived from retinoids and carotenoids, which include (a) retinal and (b) β-carotene.

Upon light absorption, 11-*cis*-retinal isomerizes to all-*trans*-retinal, which triggers a signal cascade corresponding to visualization in the cortex. Because of the integral role of vitamin A in biological processes, a deficiency in the vitamin corresponds to a plethora of diseases [42]. Notably, xerophthalmia is a group of pathologies deriving from the inability to regenerate rhodopsin and which is treated with vitamin A supplementation [45].

Reduced bioavailability of vitamin A has been shown to coincide with iron and zinc deficiency [46,47]. Bidirectionally, vitamin A supplements are reported to improve iron deficiency-associated anemia [48]. Additionally, vitamin A has emerged as a recommended supplement for improving iron absorption [49]. Cross-sectional and intervention studies point to possible intersections of iron and vitamin A in gut health and absorption, red blood cell production, and the immune response to infection [48]. The link between vitamin A and zinc status has primarily been observed in mouse models but has yet to be clearly supported in human studies; however, this has been partially attributed to the challenges of accurately measuring zinc status and deficiency in humans rather than a lack of connection [48]. Interestingly, the connection between vitamin A, iron, and zinc availability has also been observed in plant species [50], pointing to the possibility of a receptor-associated link between the three nutrients.

5.2 VITAMIN B, INCLUDING THE COBALT-CONTAINING VITAMIN B$_{12}$

Vitamin B$_{12}$ is the only vitamin that contains a metal ion and is discussed earlier in this chapter in Section 4. The other B compounds include B$_1$ (thiamine), B$_2$ (riboflavin), B$_3$ (niacin), B$_5$ (pantothenic acid), B$_6$ (pyridoxine), B$_7$ (biotin), and B$_9$ (folate) [2]. Vitamin B compounds are water-soluble, serve as enzyme cofactors, and are required for the proper functioning of most cell types in human and plant biology. Dietary consumption of all eight B vitamins is essential, as humans lack the enzymes to synthesize these compounds. In fact, not only do humans lack the biosynthetic pathways, but there is also a dearth of understanding surrounding the necessary enzymes to create vitamin B compounds. The first studies to elucidate the plant biosynthesis of vitamin B focused on thiamine (Figure 4a). Thiamine is involved in catalytic reactions as the coenzyme thiamine diphosphate [51]. Thiamine diphosphate acts as a coenzyme for transketolase, which is required for fatty acid and nucleic acid synthesis [52]. Thiamine also serves protective roles against glutamate in neurons, and as such, thiamine deficiency can present as peripheral neuritis [53]. The second vitamin B, riboflavin, is produced by plants, yeast, and prokaryotic cells, from which humans can obtain the isoalloxazine-based compound (Figure 4b) [54]. Derivatives of riboflavin, flavin mononucleotide, and flavin adenine dinucleotide serve as coenzymes for flavoproteins that participate in redox reactions [55]. Such redox reactions are required for the metabolism of energy, carbohydrates, lipids, and amino acids but may also be a potential interface with redox-active minerals like iron. Niacin, a group of compounds associated with nicotinamide, was identified in response to the pellagra outbreak in which patients experienced vitamin B_3 deficiency, resulting in dermatitis, psychological changes, and muscle weakness (Figure 4c) [56]. The spread of this disease led to in-depth research on the role of niacin compounds and their roles as NAD and NADP coenzymes. Like riboflavin, niacin coenzymes are involved in over 400 redox reactions and are famously involved in energy production as various forms of nicotinamide adenine dinucleotide (NAD, NADP, and NADPH). As such, sufficient levels of niacin are required for the maintenance of a healthy metabolism.

Vitamin B_5, or pantothenic acid, is ubiquitous in foods and is consumed through meats (e.g., chicken, beef), grains (e.g., oats), and vegetables (e.g., tomatoes, broccoli). Pantothenic acid plays roles in lipid metabolism, coenzyme A synthesis, and fatty acid synthesis (Figure 5a) [57]. Although the widespread nature of pantothenic acid in food results in few instances of deficiency [2], the rare occurrence is linked to symptoms of numbness and burning sensations of the hands and feet.

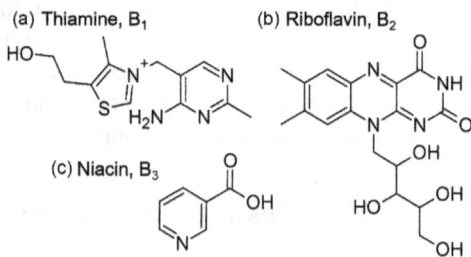

FIGURE 4   The first three vitamin B molecules derive from (a) thiamine, (b) riboflavin, and (c) niacin.

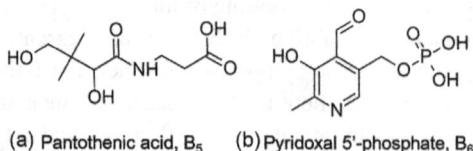

FIGURE 5   (a) Structure of vitamin B_5, also known as pantothenic acid. (b) Vitamin B_6 structures feature a pyridine-derived core.

Similar to pantothenic acid, vitamin B_6 deficiency is rare but, when present, typically results from diseases that restrict its bioavailability (Figure 5b). Due to its diverse utility, vitamin B_6 deficiency results in neurological symptoms like seizures, cardiovascular dysfunction, and dermatitis. This subclass of vitamin B_6 refers to a group of pyridine-derived compounds that share physiological functions, including the metabolism of proteins, lipids, and carbohydrates [58]. Along with their function as coenzymes, vitamin B_6 also exhibits antioxidant activity through superoxide quenching and protection against lipid oxidation.

Biotin, vitamin B_7, has one bioactive form: a bicyclic compound containing a ureido group and a tetrahydrothiophene ring (Figure 6a) [2]. Widely known for its tight binding to streptavidin, biotin is extensively used in biochemical research [59]. In human physiology, biotin serves as a coenzyme for five carboxylases involved in energy and fatty acid metabolism. Common sources of biotin include egg yolk, legumes, and nuts, and its deficiency results in a buildup of fatty and organic acids due to the disrupted metabolic pathways. Vitamin B_9, or folate, denotes a group of compounds that participate as coenzymes in the transfer of one-carbon units (Figure 6b) [60]. Commonly known for its importance during pregnancy, folic acid reduces the risk of neural tube defects and can be consumed in leafy vegetables, fruits, and legumes [61]. The methyl transfer reactions accomplished by this vitamin are essential in maintaining proper homeostasis in reactions involving DNA, RNA, lipids, proteins, and histones. Thus, folate deficiency is linked to many pathological states, including cancer, vascular disease, and developmental abnormalities. While tracking vitamin B status is challenging, there have been some documented associations between iron, B_{12}, and B_9. For instance, in cobalamin-deficiency and folate-deficiency anemia, iron deficiency is frequently observed [62,63]. However, the similarities in the symptoms of each condition can result in one masking the other, presenting challenges in treating the root cause of their simultaneous deficiencies [64,65]. While reports have observed vitamin B alterations alongside zinc deficiency or that intake of vitamin B supplements may affect mineral absorption [66–68], causal relationships remain a knowledge gap that might be worth further probing with the rise of tools for both metal monitoring and metabolomics.

(a) Biotin, B_7

(b) Folate, B_9

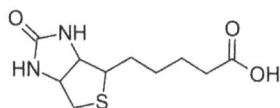
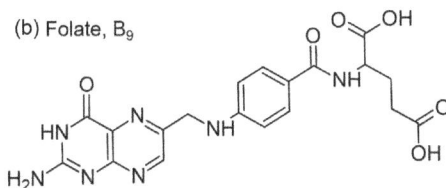

FIGURE 6 (a) Structure of vitamin B_7, commonly referred to as biotin. (b) Structure of B_9 or folate.

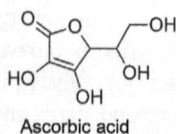

Ascorbic acid

FIGURE 7   Vitamin C, or ascorbic acid, exerts a multitude of beneficial effects on cellular function.

5.3   VITAMIN C AND IRON

Popularized by two-time Nobel laureate Linus Pauling, perhaps the most well-known vitamin is vitamin C, or ascorbic acid, which is historically famous for preventing scurvy (Figure 7) [45]. Although the amount of vitamin C required to prevent scurvy is low, the recommended dietary intake for this vitamin is much higher than that of many other vitamins. Vitamin C possesses a myriad of functions, including redox activity, catalytic activity, and antioxidant activity [69]. Importantly, this molecule acts as a cofactor for a family of biosynthetic and gene regulatory enzymes, in addition to functioning as a cofactor for the asparagyl and prolyl hydroxylases required for the downregulation of transcription factor hypoxia-inducible factor-1α [70]. Vitamin C exhibits antioxidant activity through radical scavenging and can ameliorate oxidative stress in important molecules like lipids, DNA, and proteins [71]. Behaving as a reducing agent, vitamin C activates mono- and dioxygenases required for cellular function [69]. Changes in vitamin C status are correlated to several disease states, including, but not limited to, cancer, stroke, and atherosclerosis.

Relative to the other vitamins, the relationship between vitamin C and iron is well documented, particularly with respect to the ability of the species to interact and mutually improve their bioavailability [49,72]. Vitamin C binds directly with non-heme ferric ions in acidic pH to improve iron solubility at neutral pH and adsorption, thus implicating the vitamin in improving iron bioavailability in the digestive tract [72]. For this reason, the two are frequently considered co-supplements, particularly with respect to ascorbic acid-enhancing iron supplements in iron deficiency [72–74]. More recent work has shown that the vitamin C/iron interaction may have actions and benefits beyond absorption, including modulating various iron modulatory axes such as transferrin-dependent iron uptake and reductive mechanisms [75]. Elucidating these additional relationships is warranted to fully capture the effects of nutritional intake of both micronutrients.

5.4   VITAMINS D, E, AND K

Vitamins D, E, and K have all been reported to work synergistically with mineral micronutrients, but whether the vitamins affect mineral status is less explored. Technically a misnomer, the vitamin D molecules are not strictly micronutrients, as humans can produce their precursors (Figure 8) [76]. This family is defined as steroid hormones and derivatives of a cyclopentanoperhydrophenanthrene ring system.

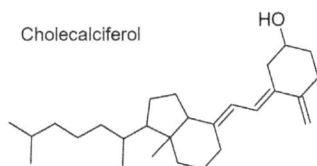

Cholecalciferol

FIGURE 8   The group of vitamin D molecules includes bioavailable cholecalciferol.

The two forms found in food and dietary supplements are vitamin D$_2$, or ergocalciferol, and vitamin D$_3$, or cholecalciferol. Both the consumed and the endogenously produced forms of vitamin D are inert and must undergo two hydroxylations to convert into their active forms [77]. The first hydroxylation occurs in the liver, and the second takes place primarily in the kidney, forming the physiologically active form of vitamin D known as calcitriol. This class of molecules is fat-soluble and helps the body maintain calcium and phosphate concentrations in serum and absorption in the gut [78]. Calcium is ubiquitous in biological functions; modulation by vitamin D is required for insulin production, cell and bone growth, and muscle function. Vitamin D deficiency can cause rickets in children and osteomalacia in adults [79]. Rickets describes a condition in which bones are not properly mineralized, leading to skeletal deformities and weak bones. The anti-rachitic properties of vitamin D compounds can be affected by age, fat malabsorption, and drug interactions. Along with calcium, vitamin D can help protect adults from osteoporosis.

Vitamin E is a group of eight molecules best known for its lipid-soluble antioxidant activity (Figure 9) [80]. Serving unique roles in different tissues, the vitamin E compounds share a chromanol core structure. A-tocopherol is the only active form of vitamin E in human biology and scavenges peroxyl radicals to prevent lipid oxidation [81]. Deficiency in vitamin E can be caused by genetic disorders such as ataxia with vitamin E deficiency, which exhibit neurological abnormalities [80]. Because of vitamin E's lipid solubility, genetic disorders that affect lipoproteins (e.g., hypobetalipoproteinemia) or fat absorption (e.g., cystic fibrosis) can result in vitamin E deficiency. Similar to most vitamin supplements, research on the long-term effects of vitamin E produces conflicting results, but a balanced diet must contain sufficient levels of α-tocopherol in order to maintain low levels of oxidative damage. Its antioxidant function could potentially serve protective functions against mineral-induced toxicity, but further studies are required to validate these claims [82].

The vitamin K class of compounds includes 2-methyl-1,4-naphthoquinone and its derivatives (Figure 10) [83]. Vitamin K compounds can be consumed

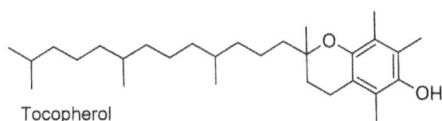

Tocopherol

FIGURE 9   Tocopherol is the only bioactive form of vitamin E in humans.

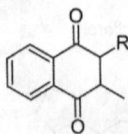

2-methyl-1,4-napthoquinone

FIGURE 10 Vitamin K and its derivatives are necessary for blood coagulation.

through legumes, leafy vegetables, and root vegetables. Luckily, vitamin K is usually consumed in excess of biological requirements, as the biochemical reactions that require this vitamin for proper enzyme function (e.g., carboxylases and reductases) play an integral role in human health [2]. In particular, vitamin K is involved in the production of prothrombin, a necessary step in blood coagulation [84]. In the rare instances of vitamin K deficiency, patients experience hypoprothrombinemia, resulting in poor blood clotting. Vitamin K and nutritional metals have shared functions, but there is no clear evidence of their direct interactions.

Each vitamin serves an integral part in maintaining proper function of the body. Treatment for diseases in which patients experience dysregulation of vitamins often includes supplementation of the required micronutrient, with recommendations stemming from observations that the adsorption of supplements can be less effective than bioavailable vitamin sources. Further understanding of formulation, vitamin-metal, and vitamin-protein interactions will provide insight into optimized treatments and nutrition recommendations.

6 METAL-BINDING NATURAL PRODUCTS IN NUTRITION

The balance of metal-containing nutrients is not solely affected by the total quantities of the minerals taken in but also by nutritional molecules, such as plant-based natural products, that can interact with metal ions. Plants have been historically used for medicinal purposes, predating modern science [85]. As such, plant metabolites have been extensively studied for their potential biochemical activity, and many drug candidates resemble compounds found in nature [86]. Thus, identification of compounds in plants that possess therapeutic activity provides a basis for the rational design of drugs. Many plant-derived compounds have therapeutic effects, understood by communities for centuries before us, as we start to understand these benefits with our modern methods. Highlighted below are two important classes of plant-derived compounds in nutrition that have been associated with metal dysregulation.

6.1 FLAVONOIDS AS METAL-BINDING NUTRIENTS

Plant-derived food products are often identified by their color or distinctive smell and taste. These characteristics are largely attributed to secondary plant metabolites, flavonoids [87]. Flavonoids are polyphenolic molecules that have a three-ring core consisting of the A and B phenyl rings joined by the central heterocyclic pyran C ring. Substitutions on this core structure divide flavonoids into subclasses: flavanols, flavanones, flavonols, flavones, anthocyanins, and isoflavones. Over 8,000 compounds fall under the flavonoid classification, with more being discovered every year [88].

While flavonoids serve multiple biological roles, they are often touted for their antioxidant activity [92,93]. The phenolic nature of flavonoids lends itself to antioxidant behavior through radical scavenging and prevention of reactive oxygen species generation. Furthermore, flavonoids can bind metal ions, potentially combating deleterious biological effects [94–96]. Redox-active metals are known to participate in Fenton or Fenton-like chemistries, resulting in the production of reactive oxygen species and oxidative stress in biological systems. The ability of flavonoids to bind reactive metal ions with varying binding affinities allows for modulation of dynamic metal populations in disease states. Flavonoids have been implicated for therapeutic effects on diseases including cancer, cardiovascular complications, neurological disorders, and metabolic pathologies, and we point the reader to the referenced reviews on these various topics [89–91].

6.2 METAL-BINDING PEPTIDES IN FOOD PRODUCTS

Plant protein hydrolysates have been isolated from a wide range of consumed plants, including soy, oat, and rice plants. The identity of peptides resulting from protein digestion depends on the employed hydrolysis method. Techniques include solvent and enzyme hydrolysis, as well as microbial fermentation [97]. The most common digestion technique is enzymatic hydrolysis using proteases like trypsin, pepsin, and pancreatin. Each enzyme cleaves at specific residues on a protein, resulting in different peptide sequences.

Peptides from plant and animal sources display therapeutic effects against human pathologies [98–100]. Providing different advantages than protein and small molecule therapeutic contenders, peptides are better able to interact with protein interfaces and cross cell membranes [101–103]. Proteins isolated from natural sources and subsequently hydrolyzed using commercially available proteases exhibit a range of therapeutic activities. These protein hydrolysates exhibit therapeutic effects toward cardiovascular, neurodegenerative, and metabolic diseases, among others [104–107]. Like their small molecule counterparts, hydrolysates have antioxidant, anticancer, and antiinflammatory activity. Due to their natural sources, plant protein hydrolysates are ideal candidates for nutraceutical applications with a lower risk of side effects compared to their synthetic analogs. The potential therapeutic efficacy can be tuned by adjusting or selecting for physical properties such as water solubility, hydrophobicity, or pH stability.

7 CONCLUSION

Bioinorganic research is rife with examples of how metals can affect the biological function of vitamins and minerals. The interplay between nutrition, disease, and metal metabolism is indeed a complex field with room for researchers from vastly different disciplines to contribute. Many questions remain as to the influence of dietary nutrients on metal status and, in particular, understanding relationships beyond observational studies of co-supplementation or co-registered deficiencies. To characterize the interactions of transition metals on human biology, it is important to differentiate whether dietary nutrients can directly coordinate with and regulate metal micronutrients, indirectly affect metal-trafficking pathways, or carry out synergistic functions with metal-containing biomolecules. The advancement in spectrophotometric tools that probe metal speciation and trafficking, including fluorescence probes and colorimetric chelators, along with the emergence of complex -omics methods, hold promise in revealing such molecular interactions between nutritional components and mineral status.

ACKNOWLEDGMENTS

This work was supported by the National Institutes of Health (NIH MIRA 5R35GM133684 and P30DK098722 to M.C.H. and the NIH MIRA 535GM1 33684-04S1 supplement to support R.L.F.) and the National Science Foundation (NSF CAREER 2048265 to M.C.H.). We also thank the Hartwell Foundation for their generous support for M.C.H. as a Hartwell Individual Biomedical Investigator, as well as the UC Davis CAMPOS Program and the University of California's Presidential Postdoctoral Fellowship for their support of M.C.H. as a CAMPOS Faculty Fellow and former UC President's Postdoctoral Fellow, respectively.

ABBREVIATIONS AND DEFINITIONS

B_1	thiamine
B_2	riboflavin
B_3	niacin
B_5	pantothenic acid
B_6	pyridoxine
B_7	biotin
B_9	folate
B_{12}	cobalamin
NAD	nicotinamide adenine dinucleotide
NAFLD	non-alcoholic fatty liver disease
EPR	electron paramagnetic resonance spectroscopy
NMR	nuclear magnetic resonance spectroscopy
UV-Vis	ultraviolet-visible absorption spectroscopy
HOMO	highest occupied molecular orbital
LUMO	lowest unoccupied molecular orbital

REFERENCES

1. A. G. Godswill, I. V. Somtochukwu, A. O. Ikechukwu, E. C. Kate, *Int. J. Food Sci.* **2020**, *3*, 1–32.
2. J. Zempleni, J. W. Suttie, J. F. Gregory lll, P. J. Stover, *Handbook of Vitamins*, 5th Ed. **2014**. https://link.springer.com/chapter/10.1007/978-3-031-08881-0_2
3. W. A. Catterall, *Voltage-Gated Calcium Channels*, CRC Press, **2022**. https://www.amazon.com/Handbook-Vitamins-Janos-Zempleni/dp/1466515562
4. O. Brzezińska, Z. Łukasik, J. Makowska, K. Walczak, *Nutrients*, **2020**, *12*, 1–22.
5. R. MacKinnon, *FEBS Lett.* **2003**, *555*, 62–65.
6. W. A. Catterall, *Physiol. Rev.* **1992**, *72*, S15–48.
7. E. E. Simon, Ed., *Hyponatremia*, Springer, 2014, pp. 256. https://books.google.com/books?id=Sd69BAAAQBAJ&source=gbs_navlinks_s
8. T. J. Jentsch, V. Stein, F. Weinreich, A. A. Zdebik, *Physiol. Rev.* **2002**, *82*, 503–568.
9. P. M. Quinton, *Nature*, **1983**, *301*, 421–422.
10. D. Kanduti, P. Sterbenk, *Mater. Soc. Med.* **2016**, *28*, 133.
11. A. J. Bird, *J. Nutr. Biochem.* **2015**, *26*, 1103–1115.
12. V. Abbate, R. Hider, *Metallomics*, **2017**, *9*, 1467–1469.
13. N. Abbaspour, R. Hurrell, R. Kelishadi, *J. Res. Med. Sci.* **2014**, *19*, 164–174.
14. W. E. Winter, L. A. L. Bazydlo, N. S. Harris, *Lab Med.* **2014**, *45*, 92–102.
15. J. M. Fernández-Real, M. Manco, *Lancet Diabet. Endocrinol.* **2014**, *2*, 513–526.
16. N. W. Solomons, *Ann. Nutr. Metabol.* **2013**, *62*, 8–17.
17. A. B. Chausmer, *J. Am. Coll. Nutr.* **1998**, *17*, 109–115.
18. G. Bjørklund, M. Dadar, L. Pivina, M. D. Doşa, Y. Semenova, J. Aaseth, *Curr. Med. Chem.* **2019**, *27*, 6643–6657.
19. D. Osman, A. Cooke, T. R. Young, E. Deery, N. J. Robinson, M. J. Warren, *Biochim. Biophys. Acta – Mol. Cell Res.* **2021**, *1868*, 118896.
20. F. O'Leary, S. Samman, *Nutrients*, **2010**, *2*, 299–316.
21. E. Nexo, E. Hoffmann-Lücke, *Am. J. Clin. Nutr.* **2011**, 1–7.
22. J. Wuerges, G. Garau, S. Geremia, S. N. Fedosov, T. E. Petersen, L. Randaccio, *Proc. Natl. Acad. Sci.* **2006**, *103*, 4386–4391.
23. L. Hannibal, V. Lysne, A.-L. Bjørke-Monsen, S. Behringer, S. C. Grünert, U. Spiekerkötter, D. W. Jacobsen, H. J. Blom, *Front. Mol. Biosci.* **2017**, *94*, 4.
24. R. A. Festa, D. J. Thiele, *Curr. Biol.* **2011**, *21*, 877–883.
25. T. Tsang, C. I. Davis, D. C. Brady, *Curr. Biol.* **2021**, *31*, R421–R427.
26. X. Ding, H. Xie, Y. J. Kang, *J. Nutr. Biochem.* **2011**, *22*, 301–310.
27. J. Chen, Y. Jiang, H. Shi, Y. Peng, X. Fan, C. Li, *Pflug. Arch. Eur. J. Physiol.* **2020**, *472*, 1415–1429.
28. C. M. Ackerman, C. J. Chang, *J. Biol. Chem.* **2018**, *293*, 4628–4635.
29. C. Gerosa, D. Fanni, T. Congiu, M. Piras, F. Cau, M. Moi, G. Faa, *J. Inorg. Biochem.* **2019**, *193*, 106–111.
30. V. Oliveri. *Coord. Chem. Rev.* **2020**, *422*, 213474.
31. Z. Tümer, L. B. Møller. *Eur. J. Hum. Gene.* **2010**, *18*, 511–518.
32. A. Członkowska, T. Litwin, P. Dusek, P. Ferenci, S. Lutsenko, V. Medici, J. K. Rybakowski, K. H. Weiss, M. L. Schilsky, *Nat. Rev. Dis. Primers.* **2018**, *4*, 1–20.
33. L. Antonucci, C. Porcu, G. Iannucci, C. Balsano, B. Barbaro, *Nutrients*, **2017**, *9*, 1–12.
34. S. L. Friedman, B. A. Neuschwander-Tetri, M. Rinella, A. J. Sanyal, *Nat. Med.* **2018**, *24*, 908–922.

35. N. H. O. Harder, B. Hieronimus, K. L. Stanhope, N. M. Shibata, V. Lee, M. V. Nunez, N. L. Keim, A. Bremer, P. J. Havel, M. C. Heffern, V. Medici, *Nutrients*, **2020**, *12*, 1–14. https://www.mdpi.com/2072-6643/12/9/2581

36. N. H. O. Harder, H. P. Lee, V. J. Flood, J. A. San Juan, S. K. Gillette, M. C. Heffern, *Front. Mol. Biosci.* **2022**, *9*, 1–13. https://pubmed.ncbi.nlm.nih.gov/35480878/

37. S. Baldari, G. D. Rocco, G. Toietta, *Int. J. Mol. Sci.* **2020**, *21*, 1–20.

38. F. Beg, M. Amrita, M. Bhatia, et al., *Int. J. Multidiscip. Curr. Res.* **2014**, 126–130. http://ijmcr.com/wp-content/uploads/2014/01/Paper21126-130.pdf

39. S. B. Bukhari, S. Memon, M. Mahroof-Tahir, M. I. Bhanger, *Spectrochim. Acta - Part A: Mol. Biomol. Spectrosc.* **2009**, *71*, 1901–1906.

40. K. T. J. Chen, M. Anantha, A. W. Y. Leung, J. A. Kulkarni, G. G. C. Militao, M. Wehbe, B. SUtherland, P. R. Cullis, M. B. Bally, *Drug Deliv. Transl. Res.* **2020**, *10*, 202–215. https://link.springer.com/article/10.1007/s13346-019-00674-7

41. A. Carazo, K. Macáková, K. Matoušová, L. Kujovská, M. Protti, P. Mladěnka, *Nutrients*, **2021**, 13, 1703.

42. M. A. Beydoun, X. Chen, K. Jha, H. A. Beydoun, A. B. Zonderman, J. A. Canas, *Nutr. Rev.* **2019**, *77*, 32–45.

43. M. Zia-ul-haq, *Carotenoids: Structure and Function in the Human Body*, Springer, **2021**. https://www.amazon.com/Carotenoids-Structure-Function-Human-Body/dp/303046458X44. K. Jomova, M. Valko, *Eur. J. Med. Chem.* **2013**, *70*, 102–110.

45. L. Rosenfeld, Vitamine-vitamin, *Clin. Chem.* **1997**, *43*, 680–685.

46. E. C. Muñoz, J. L. Rosado, P. López, H. C. Furr, L. H. Allen, *Am. J. Clin. Nutr.* **2000**, *71*, 789–794.

47. M. M. Kana-Sop, I. Gouado, M. B. Achu, J. van Camp, P. H. A. Zollo, F. J. Schweigert, D. Oberleas, T. Ekoe, *J. Nutr. Sci. Vitaminol.* **2015**, *61*, 205–214.

48. S. Y. Hess, D. I. Thurnham, R. F. Hurrell, *Influence of Provitamin A Carotenoids on Iron, Zinc, and Vitamin A Status.*. International Food Policy Research Institute (IFPRI), International Center for Tropical Agriculture (CIAT), Washington, DC, Cali, Colombia, **2005**.

49. M. A. A. López, F. C. Martos, *Int. J. Food Sci. Nutr.* **2004**, *55*, 597–606.

50. M. R. La Frano, F. F. De Moura, E. Boy, B. Lönnerdal, B. J. Burri, *Nutr. Rev.* **2014**, *72*, 289–307.

51. K. J. Carpenter, *Ann. Nutr. Metabol.* **2012**, *61*, 219–223.

52. J. Zhao, C. J. Zhong, *Neurosci. Bull.* **2009**, *25*, 94–99.

53. N. P. Staff, A. J. Windebank, *CONTIN. Lifelong Learn. Neurol.* **2014**, *20*, 1293–1306.

54. J. T Pinto, J. Zempleni, *Riboflavin* **2016**, *1*, 973–975.

55. M. Zeghouf, M. Fontecave, J. Macherel, J. Covès, *Biochem.* **1998**, *37*, 6114–6123.

56. M. A. Crook, *Nutr.* **2014**, *30*, 729–730.

57. R. B. Rucker, *Encycl. Food Health.* **2015**, 205–208.

58. M. Parra, S. Stahl, H. Hellmann, *Cells*, **2018**, *7*, 84.

59. C. M. Dundas, D. Demonte, S. Park, *Appl. Microbiol. Biotechnol.* **2013**, *97*, 9343–9353.

60. E. J. Yeo, C. Wagner, *Proc. Natl. Acad. Sci. USA*, **1994**, *91*, 210–214.

61. B. Shane, *Clin. Res. Regulat. Affairs*, **2001**, *18*, 137–159.

62. R. Carmel, *JAMA*, **1987**, *257*, 1081.

63. A. A. Zulfiqar, J. L. Pennaforte, M. Drame, E. Andrès, *Eur. J. Int. Med.* **2013**, *24*, e162–e163.

64. S. Solmaz, H. Özdoğu, C. Boğa, *Indian J. Hematol. Blood Transfus.* **2015**, *31*, 255–258.

65. R. Moll, B. Davis, *Med.* **2017**, *45*, 198–203.

66. K. Mousavi, A. Moradzadegan, *Gene Cell Tissue*, **2022**, *10*.

67. M. Horie, K. Ito, T. Hayashi, et al., *.Fujita Med. Soc.* **2017**. https://pure.fujita-hu.ac.jp/en/publications/investigation-of-blood-levels-of-zinc-vitamin-bsub12sub-and-folat

68. I. Sonmez Ozkarakaya, B. Celik, C. Karakukcu, J. Altuner Torun, *J. Trace Elem. Med. Biol.* **2021**, *65*, 126724.

69. S. J. Padayatty, A. Katz, Y. Wang, P. Eck, O. Kwon, J.-H. Lee, S. Chen, C. Corpe, A. Dutta, S. K. Dutta, M. Levine, *J. Am. Coll. Nutr.* **2003**, *22*, 18–35.

70. A. C. Carr, S. Maggini, *Nutr.* **2017**, *9*, 1–25.

71. M. Picardo, M. L. Dell'Anna, *Vitiligo*, **2010**, 231–237.

72. S. R. Lynch, J. D. Cook, *Ann. N. Y. Acad. Sci.* **1980**, *355*, 32–44.

73. A. Heffernan, C. Evans, M. Holmes, J. B. Moore, *Proc. Nutr. Soc.* **2017**, *76*, E182.

74. E. Piskin, D. Cianciosi, S. Gulec, M. Tomas, E. Capanoglu, *ACS Omega.* **2023**, *7*, 20441–20456.

75. D. J. R. Lane, D. R. Richardson, *Free Radic. Biol. Med.* **2014**, *75*, 69–83.

76. R. L. Horst, T. A. Reinhardt, G. S. Reddy, *Vitamin D*, **2005**, *1*, 15–36.

77. R. J. H. Keegan, Z. Lu, J. M. Bogusz, J. E. Williams, M. F. Holick, *Derm.-Endocrinol.* **2013**, *5*, 165–176.

78. Q. Cai, J. S. Chandler, R. H. Wasserman, R. Kumar, J. T. Penniston, *Proc. Natl. Acad. Sci. USA*, **1993**, *90*, 1345–1349.

79. M. Sahay, R. Sahay, *Indian J. Endocrinol. Metabol.* **2012**, *16*, 164.

80. E. Niki, M. G. Traber, *Ann. Nutr. Metabol.* **2012**, *61*, 207–212.

81. G. R. Buettner, *Arch. Biochem. Biophys.* **1993**, *300*, 535–543.

82. T. Miyazawa, G. C. Burdeos, M. Itaya, K. Nakagawa, T. Miyazawa, *IUBMB Life*, **2019**, *71*, 430–441.

83. G. Ferland, *Ann. Nutr. Metabol.* **2012**, *61*, 213–218.

84. M. J. Shearer, H. Bechtold, K. Andrassy, J. Koderisch, P. T. McCarthy, D. Trenk, E. Jährchen, E. Ritz, *J. Clin. Pharmacol.* **1988**, *28*, 88–95.

85. V. Seidel, *Plants*, **2020**, *9*, 1–3.

86. A. G. Atanasov, S. B. Zotchev, V. M. Dirsch, International Natural Product Sciences Taskforce, C. Supuran, *Nat. Rev. Drug Discov.* **2021**, *20*, 200–216.

87. U. Mathesius, *Plants*, **2018**, *7* (2)–30.

88. P. G. Pietta, *J. Nat. Prod.* **2000**, *63*, 1035–1042.

89. A. U. Khan, H. S. Dagur, M. Khan, N. Malik, M. Alam, M. Mushtaque, *Eur. J. Med. Chem. Rep.* **2021**, *3*, 100010.

90. H. Yi, H. Peng, X. Wu, et al., *Oxidative Med. Cell. Longev.* **2021**, **2021**. https://www.hindawi.com/journals/omcl/2021/6678662/

91. A. Ullah, S. Munir, S. L. Badshah, N. Khan, L. Ghani, B. G. Poulson, A.-H. Emwas, J. Jaremko, *Ther. Agent*, **2020**, *25*, 5243.

92. X. Fang, W. Gao, Z. Yang, Z. Gao, H. Li, *J. Agric. Food Chem.* **2020**, *68*, 6202–6211.

93. D. Zhang, L. Chu, Y. Liu, A. Wang, B. Ji, W Wu, F. Zhou, Y. Wei, Q. Cheng, S. Cai, L. Xie, G. Jia, *J. Agric. Food Chem.* **2011**, *59*, 10277–10285.

94. L. Mira, M. T. Fernandez, M. Santos, R. Rocha, M. H. Florêncio, K. R. Jennings, *Free Radic. Res.* **2002**, *36*, 1199–1208.

95. D. Malešev, V. Kuntić, *J. Serb. Chem. Soc.* **2007**, *72*, 921–939.

96. J. Ren, S. Meng, C. E. Lekka, E. Kaxiras, *J. Phys. Chem B*, **2008**, *112*, 1845–1850.

97. F. C. Wong, J. Xiao, S. Wang, K.-Y. Ee, T.-T. Chai, *Trends Food Sci. Technol.* **2020**, *99*, 44–57.

98. C. Wen, J. Zhang, H. Zhang, Y. Duan, H. Ma, *Trends Food Sci. Technol.* **2020**, *105*, 308–322.

99. C. Lammi, G. Aiello, G. Boschin, A. Arnoldi, *J. Funct. Foods*, **2019**, *55*, 135–145.

100. Y. Q. Liu, P. Strappe, W. T. Shang, Z. K. Zhou, *Crit. Rev. Food Sci. Nutr.* **2019**, *59*, 349–356.

101. P. Tavormina, B. De Coninck, N. Nikonorova, I. De Smet, B. P. A. Cammue, *Plant Cell*, **2015**, *27*, 2095–2118.
102. A. Jakubczyk, M. Karas, K. Rybczynska-Tkaczyk, E. Zielińska, D. Zieliński, *Foods*, **2020**, *9*, 846.
103. S. Datta, A. Roy, *Int. J. Pept. Res. Ther.* **2021**, *27*, 555–577.
104. M. Chalamaiah, W. Yu, J. Wu, *Food Chem.* **2018**, *245*, 205–222.
105. R. Jahanbani, S. M. Ghaffari, M. Salami, K. Vahdati, H. Sepehri, N. Namazi Sarvestani, N. Sheibani, A. A. Moosavi-Movahedi, *Plant Foods Hum. Nutr.* **2016**, *71*, 402–409.
106. A. Kuerban, A. L. Al-Malki, T. A. Kumosani, R. A. Sheikh, F. A. M. Al-Abbasi, F. A. Alshubaily, K. O. Abulnaja, S. A. Moselhy, *J. Food Biochem.* **2020**, *44*, 1–9. https://pubmed.ncbi.nlm.nih.gov/33015836/
107. R. Esfandi, W. G. Willmore, A. Tsopmo, *Foods*, **2019**, *8*, 1–12.

7 Why Is Gadolinium Still Preferred in Contrast Agents for MRI?

Mark Woods
Department of Chemistry
Portland State University
Portland, Oregon 97201, USA
Advanced Imaging Research Center
Oregon Health & Science University
Portland, Oregon 97201, USA
markw@pdx.edu

Mauro Botta
Dipartimento di Scienze e Innovazione Tecnologica
Università del Piemonte Orientale "Amedeo Avogadro"
I-15121 Alessandria, Italy
mauro.botta@uniupo.it

CONTENTS

DOI: 10.1201/9781003361756-7

ABSTRACT

For almost 40 years, complexes of gadolinium have formed a mainstay of diagnostic imaging through their use as contrast agents for magnetic resonance imaging. Once considered extremely safe, the emergence of nephrogenic systemic fibrosis in the 2000s challenged certain assumptions and practices. A feeling that the use of gadolinium in magnetic resonance imaging should be discontinued began to develop. However, alternatives have proven difficult to come by. Now some gadolinium-based agents have been removed from practice and new limitations have been introduced on how they are used. Recently, a new higher relaxivity contrast agent based on gadolinium has received approval and entered the market; another is currently in clinical trials. These developments suggest that the coordination chemistry advantages of gadolinium continue to make it the most likely candidate around which to develop newer, more effective, and safer contrast agents.

KEYWORDS

Magnetic resonance imaging; gadolinium; nephrogenic systemic fibrosis; deposition disease; relaxation agents; contrast agents

1   INTRODUCTION

To answer the question posed in the title, we must first consider what we hope to achieve by employing a contrast agent in MRI (magnetic resonance imaging). An MR image may be thought of as a nuclear magnetic resonance (NMR) experiment that primarily probes the water protons of tissue. The signals are spatially encoded by applying a gradient field that causes the water protons to resonate at different frequencies. Image contrast is achieved by means of "weighting" toward either T_1 or T_2 (the longitudinal or transverse relaxation time constants, respectively). Weighting is achieved by means of changing either the echo time or the repetition time in the acquisition sequence.

MR images are acquired using one of a number of recalled echo pulse sequences. TE is the time between the excitation pulse and the peak of the echo. TE determines how much the image is weighted toward T_2: when TE is long, magnetization in tissue with short T_2 will quickly lose coherence and not be recalled in the echo (Figure 1a). In contrast, when T_2 is long, little magnetization is lost, and the intensity of the echo is greater. In effect, a long TE allows signals

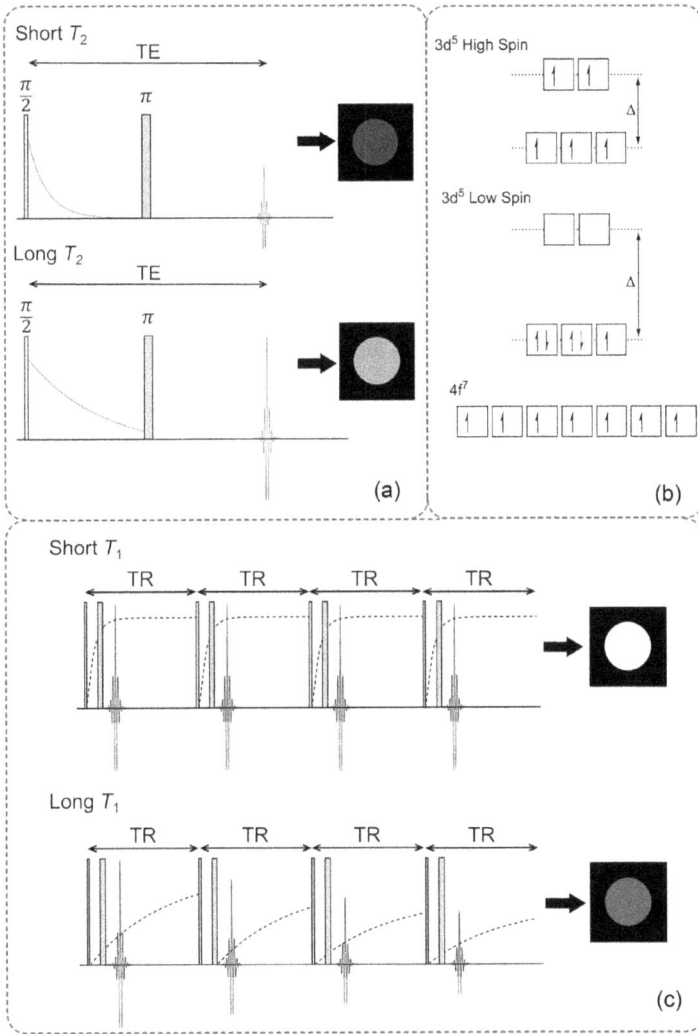

FIGURE 1 (a) The effect of a short TE on signal intensity in MR images acquired with a spin-echo pulse sequence (The dotted line represents the evolution of magnetization in the transverse plane, M_{XY}). (b) The effect of a short TR on signal intensity in an MR image acquired with a spin-echo pulse sequence (the dashed line represents the evolution of magnetization along the longitudinal axis, M_Z). When T_1 is long M_Z reaches a diminished, steady-state value prior to each excitation pulse that results in a decrease in signal intensity. (c) The distribution of electrons in the valence orbitals for $3d^5$ and $4f^7$ configurations. The degenerate 4f orbitals can be filled in only one way, but the configuration for $3d^5$ metals will depend upon the magnitude of the ligand field splitting (Δ).

in regions with short T_2 to decay while preserving signals in tissues with long T_2. A short TE will refocus most of the magnetization in all tissues, regardless of T_2.

TR is the time between successive excitation pulses and determines how much the image is weighted toward T_1 (Figure 1b). The magnitude of magnetization along the longitudinal axis (M_Z) at the time of excitation represents the maximum achievable amount of signal. If TR is long, then regardless of T_1, longitudinal equilibrium can be attained prior to the next excitation pulse and the signal intensity maximized. If TR is short, then for a tissue with a short T_1, the same situation prevails. But if T_1 is long, then recovery will be incomplete at the time of the next excitation pulse, the magnitude of M_Z will be smaller, and the signal intensity will be correspondingly weaker. Tissues with longer T_1s will appear darker. The purpose of a contrast agent is to increase the rate of water proton relaxation (shorten T_1 and T_2), permitting differentiation of tissues to which the agent has and has not been distributed.

1.1 PARAMAGNETIC MOLECULES IN MAGNETIC RESONANCE

The ability of a paramagnetic molecule to increase the rate of relaxation of water protons has been appreciated since before the first solution-state NMR experiments were even performed. Felix Bloch and his team were the first to conduct a solution-state NMR experiment [1], but while conducting this groundbreaking work, they had little sense of how long it would take the water protons in their sample to return to equilibrium. At this distance from their experiments, it seems almost amazing that, even before they had conducted their experiments and without knowing how long T_1 might be, they were fully aware that a paramagnetic solute could be used to shorten T_1 [1,2]. The very first solution-state magnetic experiment employed a relaxation agent! 25 years later the very first MRI experiment also employed a paramagnetic manganese salt to shorten T_1 and reduce the total acquisition time [3].

Relaxation in an NMR experiment occurs when the dipole of the water proton experiences the local magnetic field produced by another dipole, such as another water proton. Because molecules are not static (they translate, rotate, and vibrate), this local magnetic field oscillates, and in doing so, it applies torque to the dipole of the water proton. The orientation of the water proton dipole with respect to the primary magnetic field (B_0) is altered. Over the sum of all spins and over time, the effect of these dipole–dipole interactions is to return the sample to equilibrium in both the longitudinal and transverse dimensions. Relaxation is a bulk and not a molecular property in NMR.

Because the magnetic moments of nuclei are small and dipole–dipole interactions are very distance-dependent (to the inverse sixth power), relaxation is slow in this situation. But the magnetic moment of an unpaired electron is very large, which means that it can have a much larger effect on the water proton dipole. Clearly, more unpaired electrons will be better than fewer, so a metal ion that has multiple unpaired electrons is a strong candidate to serve as a relaxation agent. But relaxation depends on more than just having a large oscillating field; the frequency of oscillation is also important. Relaxation is most effective when the frequency of oscillation is close to the proton Larmor frequency [4]. In a diamagnetic system, the frequency of oscillation is the rate at which the molecule tumbles ($1/\tau_R$), but in a paramagnetic system, the rate of tumbling combines with that of electron spin relaxation ($1/T_{1e}$ and $1/T_{2e}$). Electron spin relaxation is generally rapid, faster than ideal for catalyzing the relaxation of water protons. This is especially true in multielectron systems, where interelectron interactions promote faster electron spin relaxation. Thus, metal ions that have symmetrical, singly filled valence shells and thus the least interelectronic interactions will have the slow electron spin relaxation characteristics demanded for effective relaxation agents.

1.2   WHY WAS GADOLINIUM USED IN FIRST PLACE?

It follows from the proceeding that of the 90 stable, naturally occurring elements only three are likely candidates for making a highly effective relaxation agent: Mn^{2+} (d^5), Fe^{3+}(d^5), and Gd^{3+}(f^7) (Figure 1c). And this only if Mn^{2+} and Fe^{3+} are in a high-spin state. From this list, the choice of gadolinium as the basis for the first generation of contrast agents may seem surprising, but it was in fact logical. Several considerations factor into whether an agent will be safe and effective.

1.2.1   Safe and Soluble

Using metal ions in any *in vivo* application presents two challenges. The first of which is quite simple: most metal ions are not freely soluble in water at pH 7.4. The Lewis acidic nature of metals causes deprotonation of water, which leads to formation of complex hydroxide gels which precipitate from solutions at higher pHs (Figure 2a). This problem can be remedied by wrapping the metal ion in a polydentate ligand (Figure 2b and c) that reduces the Lewis acidity of the metal ion and prevents the formation of complex hydroxide gels.

The second challenge is the inherent toxicity of metal ions. This statement may seem surprising given that many metal ions are essential minerals without which life could not exist. However, this does not mean that these essential minerals are without potential toxic effects. This is a subject to which we will return later in this discussion. But at this stage, we can simply note that xenobiotic metal ions, those that do not naturally occur in biological systems (in this case, gadolinium), have chemistries that are incompatible with those of the biological system. They can interfere with normal biological function. Metals that are essential minerals have specifically evolved systems for the accumulation, transport, storage, and use of the ions [5]. These systems tightly regulate these metals in the body so that almost none of them can be found floating freely in solution in the body [5]. This avoids adverse reactions and potential toxic effects, but if these systems are overwhelmed, the toxic effects of even these essential minerals can be severe. This means that any metal ion used in a diagnostic must be administered in the form of a stable chelate.

Chelation means that many, or even all, of the coordination sites of the metal ion are occupied by a single polydentate ligand. The chelate effect stabilizes a complex by increasing the entropy of the system. It also shields the metal ion from its surroundings, often even changing its charge (Figure 2b). It is essential that any metal ion used as a contrast agent be robustly chelated by a polydentate ligand. This ligand will both keep the metal ion in solution and keep it safe by minimizing interactions with the biological medium.

1.2.1.1   Chelate Stability

It seems like a simple matter to say that the metal chelate must be stable; after all, the major safety concern is the possibility of releasing the central metal ion from the

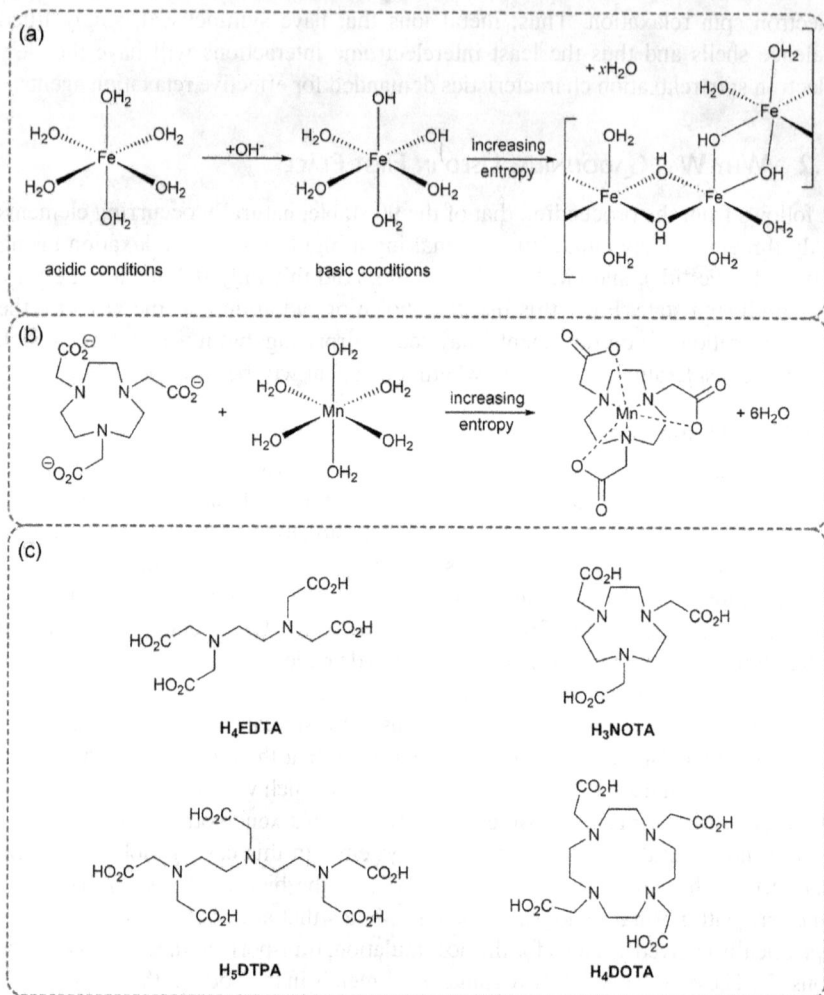

FIGURE 2 (a) The Lewis acidity of metal ions produces high molecular weight metal hydroxide gels, limiting the solubility of metal ions at higher pH. (b) The chelate effect is entropy driven, the seven species on the right of the equation represent a more disordered state than the two on the left. (c) The structures of four common polydentate aminocarboxylate ligands widely used to chelate transition metal (top) and lanthanides (bottom).

agent into the body. But it is important to be clear about what we mean by "stable". Stability is defined by a stability constant (K_{ML}), an equilibrium constant that quantifies the ratio of the amount of metal that is retained in the ligand and that which has escaped the ligand at equilibrium (Equation 1). On the basis that the primary safety concern with any contrast agent is the release of the metal ion in the body, K_{ML} appears to be a straightforward measure of safety, but such an analysis is incorrect. After administration, a contrast agent never reaches chemical equilibrium. So K_{ML} does not provide an indication of how much Gd^{3+} may be released into the body after administration of a contrast agent. Despite this, it is quite common for scientific articles published in the last 20 or so years to categorize contrast agents into (less stable) linear agents and (more stable) macrocyclic agents based on differences in the stability constants of these agents.

$$K_{\mathrm{ML}} = \frac{[\mathrm{ML}]}{[\mathrm{M}][\mathrm{L}]} \tag{1}$$

The extent to which a contrast agent will release its metal ion into the body depends not on thermodynamic factors but on kinetics [6]. It is the relative rates of clearance and dissociation that are important in determining safety. If an agent is excreted more quickly than it dissociates, then it will release very little metal into the body and can be considered safe. Conversely, an agent that is excreted more slowly than it dissociates would be expected to release larger quantities of metal into the body and would be viewed as less safe. So, unless a contrast agent is to be retained in the body for a longer than usual period, the primary consideration with respect to its safety is the kinetics of dissociation. However, this aspect of a contrast agent's behavior is harder to characterize. Whereas thermodynamic stability is well described by a single constant (K_{ML}) that can readily be compared with other constants, a rate constant for dissociation varies depending on the conditions under which it was measured. This means that a measurement made for one gadolinium-based contrast agent may not be directly comparable with that of another. Compounding this problem, the actual *in vivo* mechanism of dissociation is itself a matter of disagreement [7]. Various mechanisms for dissociation have been advanced, such as trans-metallation, proton-mediated dissociation and spontaneous dissociation. But both endogenous metals ions and protons are available only at concentrations of 10^{-8} M or below in physiological fluids. Spontaneous dissociation of the chelate may be the most relevant *in vivo* but is difficult to quantify. In the absence of a consensus on the mechanism of dissociation, it is perhaps not surprising that there is no universally accepted set of conditions under which dissociation should be measured.

The significance of this distinction can be seen from Table 1, in which two contrast agents currently in clinical use are compared (Figure 3). The linear GdDTPA appears to be slightly more stable than the macrocyclic GdDO3A-butrol, but the dissociation data tell a different story. Comparing these data, it is evident that the macrocyclic chelate is in fact the more robust chelate. And this conclusion is supported by the clinical observations discussed later. A thorough review of the factors that influence the kinetic robustness of a chelate was published by Long and co-workers [7].

When a contrast agent is administered, it is far from equilibrium; there is little or no liberated metal present, and if an ion is liberated, it is insoluble in physiological fluids and is quickly removed from the system. Le Châtelier's principle will continue to push the contrast agent toward the release of more and more metal. So even the most stable contrast agent will leak a small amount of metal into the body; the extent depends upon how quickly the agent is excreted from the body.

TABLE 1

A Comparison of Thermodynamic and Kinetic Properties of a Linear Contrast Agent – Gadopentate (GdDTPA) and a Macrocyclic Contrast Agent – Gadobutrol (GdDO3A-Butrol). It is Evident That the Linear Agent Registers a Slightly Higher Stability Constant (K_{ML}) than the Macrocyclic Agent Suggesting Comparable Safety Profiles. But It Is the Rate of Dissociation (k_D) Measured in 0.1 M HCl That Is the Relevant Parameter and Here the Macrocyclic Chelate Is Found to Release the Gd^{3+} Two Orders of Magnitude More Slowly

	Gadopentate	Gadobutrol
$\log K_{GdL}$	22.2	21.8
k_D/s^{-1}	1.2×10^{-3}	2.8×10^{-5}

1.2.1.2 Rate of Excretion

From the preceding, it follows that clearance should be as rapid as possible. Once the imaging protocol is complete, there is no reason for the agent to remain in the body. Indeed, the longer it remains in the body, the more likely it is that an adverse reaction (namely metal ion release) will occur. There are two primary routes by which foreign substances can be eliminated from the body: biliary (liver) and renal (kidney) clearance. By far the most rapid of these is renal clearance. Furthermore, renal clearance occurs through a simple filtration process, removing small solutes from the blood; no enzymes are involved to modify the structure of the substance. It is best if a contrast agent undergoes rapid renal clearance.

This puts a restriction on the size of the contrast agent. An important study by Brechbiel and workers used dendrimers of different generations to carefully control the size of contrast agents and monitor how this influenced the rate and extent of renal clearance [8]. This showed that for dendrimers below generation 4 (G4), the rate of renal clearance was unaffected by size. But above G4, the clearance rate began to be compromised. To ensure safety, a contrast agent should be small and hydrophilic so that it can be efficiently cleared through the kidneys before metal ion release can occur.

1.2.2 An Effective Relaxation Agent

The theory of paramagnetic relaxation was developed in the early days of NMR and was described in a series of papers by Solomon, Bloembergen, and Morgan [9–11]. This theory tells us that, in addition to the slow electron spin relaxation characteristics provided by these metal ions, three other parameters govern the effectiveness of a contrast agent, which is called the agent's relaxivity. The increase in the water proton relaxation rate constant generated by a 1 mM concentration of the agent.

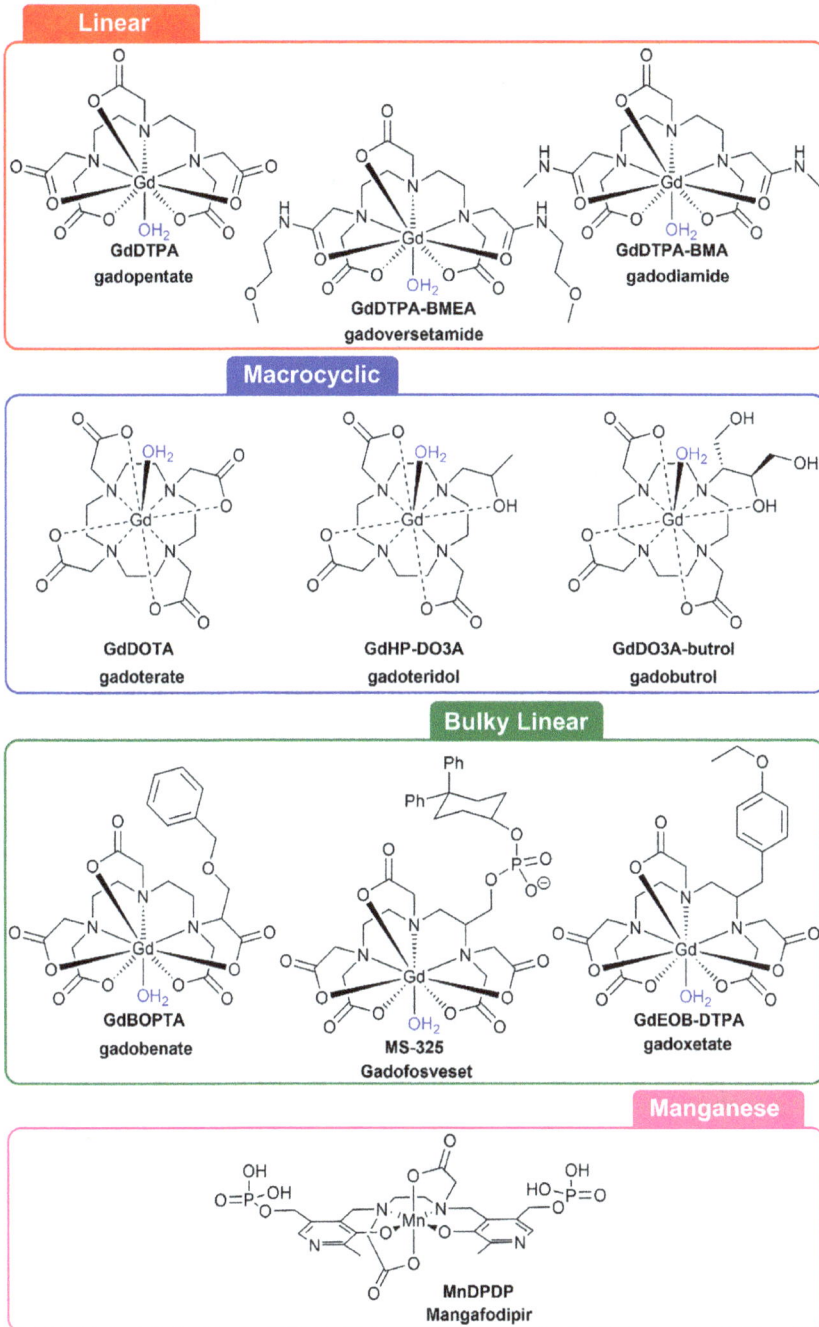

FIGURE 3 The structures (by conventional classification) of MRI contrast agents with world-wide approval for clinical use or in clinical trials in the early 2000s.

1.2.2.1   The Number and Position of Water Molecules (q/r^{-6})

From the preceding discussion, it is evident that any paramagnetic species will be most effective the closer the water proton is to the paramagnetic metal ion. The closest the water molecule can come to the metal center is to chemically bond with it. If a water molecule bound to the metal ion exchanges rapidly with those of the bulk solvent, then the entire solvent will experience the presence of the paramagnetic ion. This "inner-sphere" mechanism is the most important mechanism in the paramagnetic relaxation of water protons. The number of water molecules bound to the metal ion is denoted as q, and their distance from the metal ion is denoted as r. q and r are often treated as independent parameters, but they should really be considered as a single parameter representing the overall hydration of the metal ion [12,13]. Relaxivity scales linearly with q, so increasing the number of bound water molecules will lead to higher relaxivity. However, q cannot be increased without limit; for every additional coordinated water molecule, the chelating ligand must decrease its denticity by one. It is evident from Figure 2b that this will reduce the stability of the contrast agent, so a compromise must be reached between chelate stability and relaxivity.

For Gd^{3+}, the balance point for this compromise is comparably easy to identify. Gd^{3+} typically adopts coordination numbers (CN) between 8 and 10; with the polyaminocarboxylate ligands commonly employed in contrast agents, CN=9 is by far the most common. An octadentate ligand is usually sufficient to robustly chelate the Gd^{3+} ion, leaving one vacant coordination site that can be occupied by water. Figure 3 shows the structures of the contrast agents that were available for clinical use in most markets at some point between 2000 and 2020. Notably, all the Gd^{3+}-based agents have $q = 1$.

The balance point for Mn^{2+} and Fe^{3+} chelates is much harder to identify. Because these ions are more typically CN=6 (although CN=7 is possible), the potential "cost" of giving up denticity is higher than for gadolinium. Opening coordination for water access can lead to more labile chelates.

1.2.2.2   The Rate of Water Exchange $(1/\tau_M)$

It is critical that any coordinated molecules exchange with those of the bulk solvent rapidly. Because a coordinated water molecule is very close to the paramagnetic ion, it feels the effect of the oscillating magnetic field very strongly. There is no need for it to reside on the metal for a long time for its nuclear dipole to be reoriented. Fast water exchange ensures that many more water molecules experience the effect of the paramagnet, increasing the overall effect on water T_1. The Solomon–Bloembergen–Morgan theory can be used to calculate the optimal exchange rate constant (Figure 4).

1.2.2.3   The Rate of Tumbling $(1/\tau_R)$

A low-molecular-weight chelate tumbles quickly in solution $(\tau_R < 100$ ps). At this rate, the dipole–dipole interaction oscillates at about two orders of magnitude more quickly than the Larmor frequency of the water proton. The efficiency of the agent can be improved if the frequency of tumbling is made slower. This is easy

$\Delta^2 = 6.8 \times 10^{-18}$ s^{-2}, $\tau_V = 25$ ps, *e.g.* **GdDOTFA**

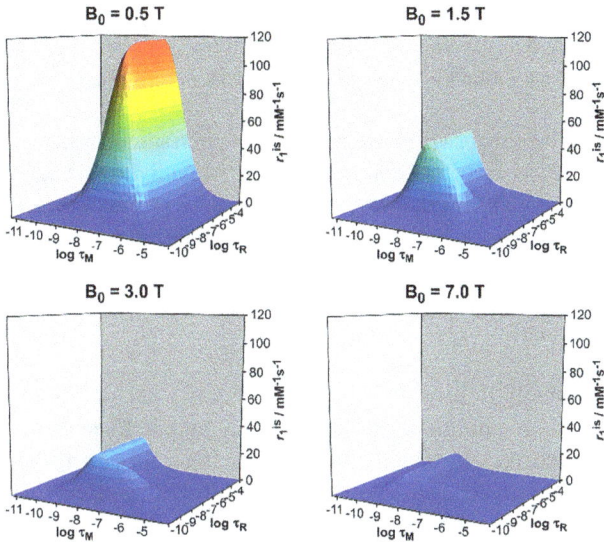

$\Delta^2 = 1.6 \times 10^{-19}$ s^{-2}, $\tau_V = 7.7$ ps, *e.g.* **GdDOTA**

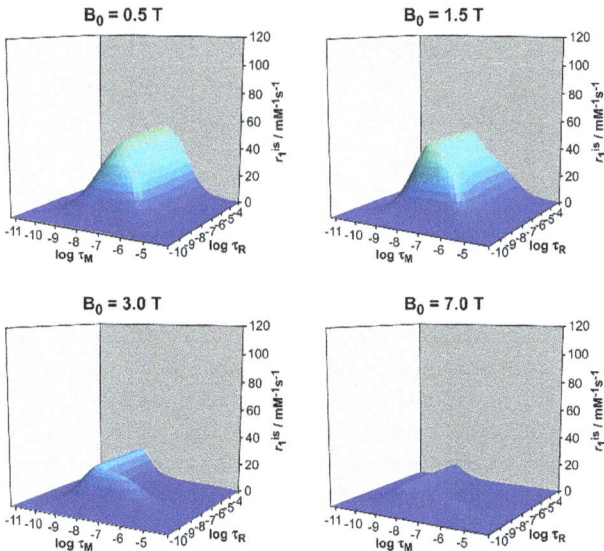

FIGURE 4 Calculations of the relaxivity as a function of water exchange (τ_M) and molecular tumbling (τ_R) for two $q=1$ gadolinium chelates at different magnetic field strengths. (a) Calculated using the electron spin relaxation characteristics of a typical macrocyclic chelate such as GdDOTA: $\Delta^2 = 1.6 \times 10^{-19}$ s^{-2}, $\tau_V = 7.7$ ps. (b) Calculated using the electron spin relaxation characteristics of an optimal chelate such as GdDOTFA: $\Delta^2 = 6.8 \times 10^{-18}$ s^{-2}, $\tau_V = 25$ ps.

to achieve – it has long been known that larger molecules tumble more slowly in solution than small ones. The simple expedient of making the contrast agent bigger, or coupling it to a larger macromolecule, will have the desired effect. This is also found through a quantitative analysis of the Solomon–Bloembergen–Morgan theory (Figure 4).

The perceptive reader will have noticed the contradiction that has now arisen. By increasing the size of the contrast agent, its relaxivity will increase, making it a better relaxation agent. However, this change in size will affect other critical aspects of the contrast agent's performance, specifically how and how quickly it is cleared from the body. This has significant implications for the agent's safety. The change in size may also have an impact on the agent's pharmacokinetics, as we shall see shortly.

1.2.3 Pharmacokinetics

Contrast agents are administered intravenously and so to enter tissue they must pass through the narrow endothelial gap junctions that form the blood vessel walls. Unsurprisingly, chelate size will have a substantial effect on how the agent extravasates; larger agents can find themselves confined to the vasculature and effectively become blood pool agents. This can be an excellent result if angiography is the goal, but for almost any other application, this is extremely detrimental. Furthermore, smaller agents are also preferred for rapid renal clearance; both of these factors point to a need for low-molecular-weight chelates.

1.3   Clinical Contrast Agents Then and Now

Gd^{3+} has formed the basis of all but one of the contrast agents approved for worldwide clinical use since 1983. Although Gd^{3+} has seven unpaired electrons, more than either Mn^{2+} or Fe^{3+}, high-spin Mn^{2+} typically has longer electron spin relaxation characteristics and is potentially a more effective relaxation agent. But none of these metal ions will significantly outperform the others as a relaxation agent if the chelate remains small and in the fast water exchange regime. It is unlikely that either Mn^{2+} or Fe^{3+} can accommodate more water molecules than Gd^{3+} and retain adequate robustness.

The reasons for the use of Gd^{3+} really center around its coordination chemistry. Gd^{3+} forms coordination bonds with its ligands that are primarily electrostatic in nature. It is a strong Lewis acid, so these bonds can be quite strong. This means that a robust chelate can be obtained if some simple principles of coordination chemistry are followed:

- The ligand should maximize denticity. For Gd^{3+}, this can be achieved (CN=8) while still leaving one coordination site open for water.
- Gd^{3+} is a hard acid, so hard bases, such as oxygen, should be used as donor atoms.
- Gd^{3+} is a large metal ion, so five-membered chelate rings are preferred.
- The chelate will be more robust if the ligand is pre-organized, which means that its conformation in the chelate is the same as its lowest energy conformation.

- The ligand should be polyanionic. This will mask the positive charge of the metal and also create stronger electrostatic interactions.
- The ligand should be macrocyclic.

Polyaminocarboxylate ligands are excellent for gadolinium. The large number of coordination sites available on Gd^{3+} means that it can be bound tightly by an octadentate polyaminocarboxylate ligand while leaving one coordination site open for water. For a relaxation agent, this is an advantageous situation because the inner-sphere mechanism can operate as effectively as possible without compromising safety.

There is no need to worry about geometry or ligand fields. The 4f orbitals of its valence shell are not involved in bonding and experience only very weak ligand fields. The 4f orbitals are always degenerate (Figure 1c), meaning that they are always singly occupied. The coordination geometry in a Gd^{3+} chelate is determined by the conformational properties of the ligand. There is no ligand field stabilization energy to consider, and so a wide range of polyaminocarboxylate ligands can easily be applied to creating robust chelates. The first contrast agent to enter clinical use was GdDTPA, using effectively an "off-the-shelf" ligand (Figures 2 and 3).

2 PROBLEMS WITH THE USE OF GADOLINIUM IN MRI

Contrast agents first went into clinical trials in 1983 and were widely used, almost without incident, for the next 25 years. These contrast agents would be classified as among the safest pharmaceuticals, with the most common adverse effect being rare instances of anaphylaxis [14]. Prior to 2000, numerous studies were published [15] demonstrating the superior safety profile of contrast agents for MRI in comparison to the iodinated agents used in computed tomography (CT): lower incidence of anaphylaxis, better kidney tolerance, etc.. But this apparently excellent safety profile may have directly contributed to the emergence of problems.

2.1 NEPHROGENIC SYSTEMIC FIBROSIS (NSF)

By the late 1990s, contrast agents based on gadolinium were considered so safe that one may describe the attitude toward their use as complacent. One such example is the apparently routine use of doses several times higher than the approved 0.1 mmol/kg in the development of MR angiography techniques in the late 1990s [16]. This type of off-label use of contrast agents was at the time not regarded as problematic or unduly risky in this period. Mostly *because* problems with this class of pharmaceuticals were so rare.

But problems were looming, and when they emerged, they forever changed attitudes toward and the practice of MRI with contrast agents. Around the turn of the century, some patients presented with hard or swollen lesions on their skin, leading to the name: nephrogenic fibrosing dermopathy (Figure 5a) [17,18]. It was not long before this fibrosing was found to occur not just in the skin but also in the internal organs. The condition was renamed NSF [19,20]. Two factors appeared to relate to all sufferers: they had recently received a contrast-enhanced MRI, and

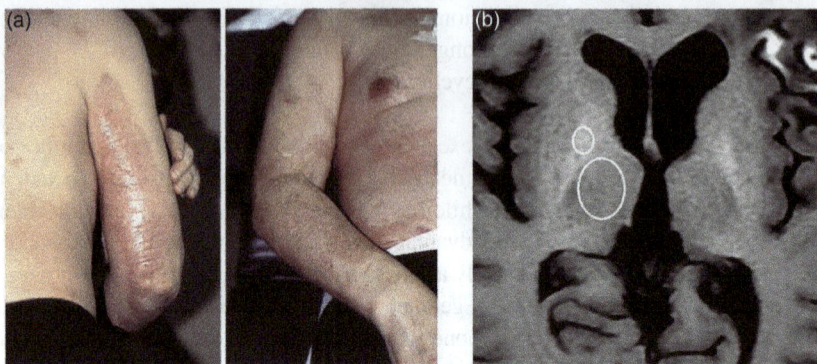

FIGURE 5 (a) Photographs of the lesions caused by NSF. (b) A T_1-weighted MR image of the human brain showing regions of hyperintensity in the dentate nucleus.

they had some degree of kidney failure. It became apparent and is now widely accepted that somehow gadolinium was causing NSF.

NSF was a very serious condition; the hard-fibrosed lesions could be painful and progress throughout the body. On the skin, they tended to appear on the limbs and could prevent joints from functioning. On internal organs, they could eventually lead to organ damage. Some patients eventually died from the condition. But NSF was limited; the only patients who contracted it were those who had pre-existing kidney failure, a group of patients often in need of contrast-enhanced MRI scans. The full extent of NSF may never be truly known, but at its height, one estimate puts the number of lawsuits related to NSF higher than the number of sufferers.

In response to NSF, the radiological community developed a sudden interest in the chemistry of contrast agents, which, had it occurred earlier, may have prevented NSF from occurring in the first place. The literature of the first decade of the 2000s is abundant with descriptions of contrast agents and their characteristics, such as stability, *in vivo* half-life, etc. [20]. One of the most common distinctions made at this time was between the linear agents derived from DTPA and the macrocyclic agents derived from DOTA. It would come as no surprise to the coordination chemist that, when the agent used could be identified, cases of NSF were found to almost exclusively have occurred after administration of a linear contrast agent. No unconfounded instance of a sufferer receiving a macrocyclic agent was confirmed. One agent in particular was strongly associated with incidents of NSF: the linear GdDTPA-BMA. Although this was a widely used contrast agent, there were many in the chemistry community who felt that this agent was insufficiently robust and should not have been approved in the first place. The rationale for why this agent was acceptable for *in vivo* applications was based primarily on thermodynamic rather than kinetic considerations and assumptions about *in vivo* chemistry that may not be valid [21].

In response to the emergence of NSF, regulatory bodies took action, prohibiting the use of contrast media in patients with renal failure and, in some cases, revoking the approvals of some linear agents. GdDTPA-BMA is no longer available as a contrast agent in the UK and much of the European Union.

The analogous GdDTPA-BMEA was purchased from Mallinckrodt by Guerbet, who immediately removed it from the market. There are fewer contrast agents available today than there were during the emergence of NSF (Figure 6). There is also widespread acceptance that not all contrast agents are the same and that macrocyclic agents are generally safer. It is noteworthy that during this time, the only

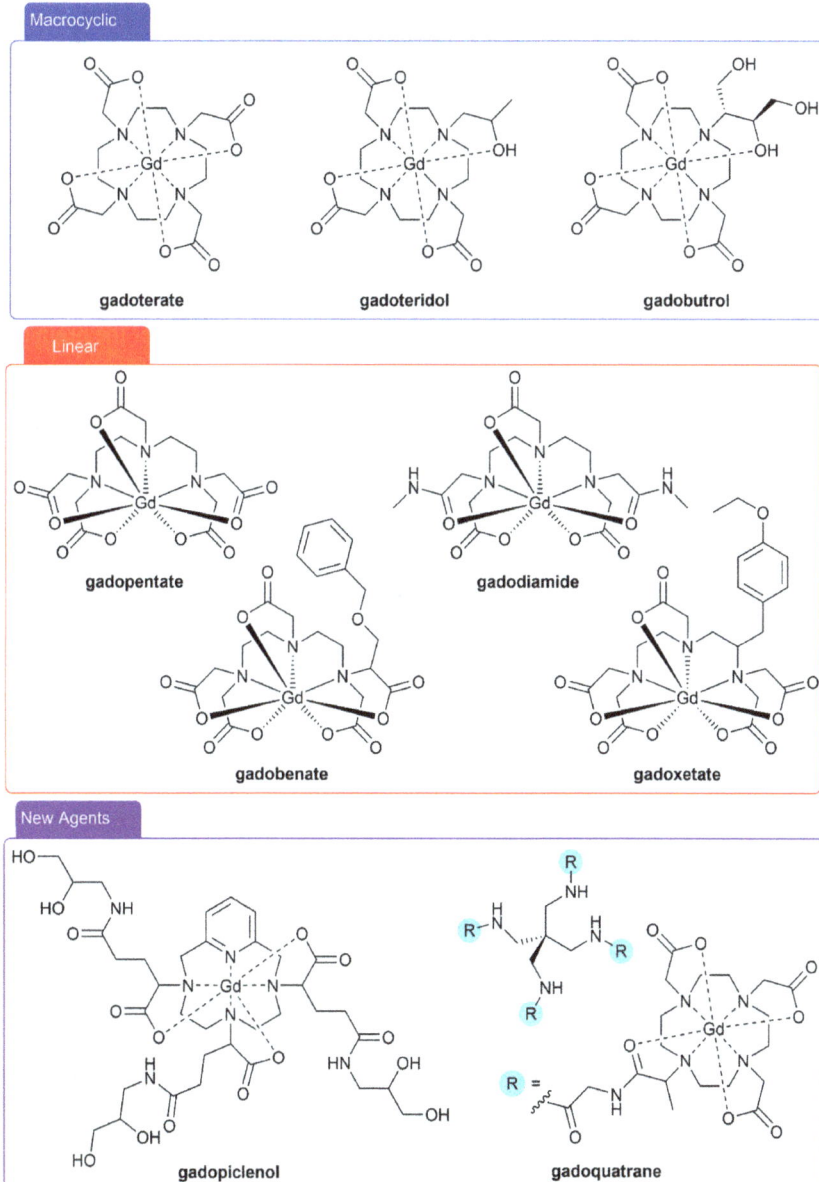

FIGURE 6   The structures of MRI contrast agents with world-wide approval for clinical use or in clinical trials at the time of writing.

available non-gadolinium agent, MnDPDP, was also removed from the market. In the noise about gadolinium and NSF, it was not widely noted, and although commercial reasons were often cited, there were also concerns over its safety [22].

2.2 BRAIN DEPOSITION

Based on the work of Tweedle and co-workers [23–25], it was believed that contrast agents did not cross the tight endothelial gap junctions of the blood-brain barrier. And it is true to say that contrast agents are largely excluded from the brain except where vascular integrity is compromised. So, the radiological community was startled when, in 2014, Kanda and co-workers reported higher than normal signal intensities in the dentate nucleus and globus pallidus on T_1-weighted, non-contrast–enhanced MR scans of patients who had previously undergone at least six contrast-enhanced MR exams (Figure 5b) [26]. The authors attributed this hyperintensity to the possible presence of gadolinium in these regions of the brain. Although the blood-brain barrier of many of these patients may have been compromised, this report nonetheless raised serious questions about how much gadolinium could enter the brain and whether another problem with contrast agents existed.

The science around gadolinium brain deposition remains hard to understand; there is a paradox here that is hard to resolve. MR images show hyperintensity in certain parts of the brain, such as the dentate nucleus. Other studies find gadolinium in the same parts of the brain. But this case is far from closed. To influence signal intensity in an MR image, gadolinium must be in solution; *ergo*, it must be in the form of an intact chelate because the liberated metal is insoluble and cannot influence signal intensity. But studies, such as a comparison of linear and macrocyclic agents, point to liberated metal accumulating in these parts of the brain. If this is so, then it should have no effect on the MR image. So, which is it? Is the agent intact but trapped in the brain? Or has the metal ion escaped and been mineralized in the brain? This is a significant difference, because if it is the former, then it is likely that there are no safety implications. But if it is the latter, then there may be cause for concern. These two seemingly irreconcilable observations are not yet understood. Whatever the situation, to date, there are no known clinical symptoms associated with the accumulation of gadolinium in the brain.

2.3 GADOLINIUM DEPOSITION DISEASE

We will not dwell for long on the subject of "gadolinium deposition disease," but we cannot simply pass over the subject. The reader is directed to an excellent review [27] and an equally thorough opinion piece [28] for a detailed analysis. Malikova makes the following important observation about the origins of "gadolinium deposition disease."

> *...their results were based on questioning the anonymous participates[sic] from "MRI-Gadolinium-Toxicity Support Group", which is a group of patients, their friends and families active on social networks.*

In short, this "disease" originates from questioning those who have already attributed adverse health effects (from which they genuinely suffer) not to a disease or some other factor but definitively to a contrast-enhanced MRI exam. The conclusion seems to have preceded the evidence! In a retrospective effort to find evidence, it has become common practice to repeatedly administer extremely high doses of a contrast agent to animal models. The reason for this is that the amount of residual gadolinium in the body 24 hours after a contrast-enhanced MRI is extremely low [23]. And of that, most accumulate first in the liver before finally being deposited in bone [24,29]. Even with the high sensitivity of modern ICP-MS (inductively coupled plasma – mass spectrometry), it is hard to detect residual gadolinium in other tissues. Administering multiple high doses could increase the levels of residual gadolinium in these other tissues, making it detectable. The problem is that this approach overwhelms the body's systems with contrast agents. The kidneys cannot filter the agent from the blood as quickly, meaning longer circulation times. Not only will there be more liberated gadolinium because the dose was higher, but a greater proportion of the dose will lose its gadolinium. Because gadolinium is xenobiotic, there are no proteins or pathways specifically evolved to manage its presence *in vivo*. We speculate that gadolinium enters pathways used to manage endogenous metal ions, with some pathways predominating over others depending upon the similarity of the chemistry of the endogenous ion with that of gadolinium. As the levels of liberated gadolinium become vastly elevated, lower affinity pathways are more likely to be exploited by gadolinium. The distribution and behavior of gadolinium under these conditions will not be reflective of the situation that prevails in clinical practice. We choose not to cite examples of this practice here, but caution the reader that in the current climate, any study into the possible side effects of gadolinium needs to be carefully evaluated in the context of experimental design and the likely applicability of the results to the typical use patterns of contrast agents in a clinical setting.

"Gadolinium deposition disease" is a vague condition with a wide range of seemingly unrelated symptoms. The recognized symptoms of this "disease" include: burning sensation in the arms or legs, tightness of hands or feet, joint/bone pain, head/neck pain, mental confusion/brain fog, skin discoloration, skin thickening, persistent headaches, vision problems, hearing problems, hair loss, itchy skin, nausea, diarrhea, vomiting, and breathing problems. It is unclear how the low levels of liberated gadolinium that are present after a contrast-enhanced MRI can cause this wide range of symptoms. This is not to say that there is no suffering; these patients' symptoms are real. But there is a real risk in blindly attributing them to deposited gadolinium. Some providers have begun to advocate chelation therapy to remove deposited gadolinium. There are two important points to make regarding this suggestion. (1) Not only might chelation therapy not address the underlying cause of the condition, but it may also distract from more appropriate treatments. There is, as yet, no definitive evidence that gadolinium is the causative agent of these symptoms, chelation therapy may be an attempt to treat a cause that is not actually the cause. After all, it is well known that liberated gadolinium begins to mineralize in bone shortly after administration [23,24].

Much (most?) of the residual gadolinium will quickly become unavailable for removal by chelation therapy. (2) Chelation therapy is also potentially dangerous. In life-threatening situations, such as lead poisoning or iron overload, chelation therapy can be necessary. However, the side effects can be serious, and it is not a treatment to be undertaken lightly.

2.4 SUMMARY

Contrast agents based on gadolinium have been widely used with very few adverse events. However, the strength of their safety profile led to a culture in which the very real risks of the use of these agents were not adequately respected. The administration of these agents to renally compromised patients was almost inevitably going to lead to problems. This issue was compounded by a lack of awareness that not all agents were equivalent, and some arguably should never have been approved for clinical use. Since the emergence of NSF restrictions on the use of contrast agents and linear agents specifically have reduced adverse events.

3   ALTERNATIVES TO GADOLINIUM

It is not surprising that, in light of the concerns about the safety of gadolinium described in Section 2, interest grew in the possibility of finding an alternative to this xenobiotic metal ion [30]. Both Mn^{2+} and Fe^{3+} have been investigated, but, thus far, without progress into clinical practice.

3.1   IRON(III)

One of the most often cited arguments in favor of replacing gadolinium with iron is that iron is an essential mineral. This is often erroneously taken to mean that iron has no toxic effects on the body. On the contrary, iron can be extremely detrimental to health despite being an essential mineral. It is estimated that more than a million people in the United States alone suffer from hemochromatosis, or iron overload [31]. The body has no mechanism for excreting iron because iron is an extremely scarce nutrient. When the levels of iron present in the body overwhelm the systems that handle it, a range of adverse reactions occur, such as arrythmia and heart failure, liver problems such as cirrhosis, cancer and even liver failure, arthritis, diabetes, and damage to or even failure of other organs such as the spleen, adrenal glands, pituitary gland, gallbladder, or thyroid. These conditions can ultimately lead to death.

The damage caused by iron is generally the result of its redox chemistry and yet the value of iron in biological systems is its redox chemistry that allows hemoglobin, myoglobin, and iron sulfur clusters, among others, to function. But this redox chemistry can also be extremely damaging, producing reactive oxygen species and damaging the integrity of tissue and cells. In the case of iron, the capacity of the body to sequester and manage a small amount of liberated metal ion is substantial *if* iron is already well regulated. But for many individuals, this situation may not prevail.

3.2 MANGANESE(II)

The arguments in favor of Mn^{2+} are slightly different, despite manganese also being an essential mineral. Manganese may exhibit the slowest electron spin relaxation of any element; in principle, Mn^{2+} may make for the most effective relaxation agent possible. But an excess of manganese may be equally dangerous: manganism (manganese overload) is less common and is most usually associated with metal workers such as welders and machinists. Manganism is a neurological condition with symptoms similar to those of Parkinson's disease, and since the endogenous levels of manganese are much lower than those of iron, and the body's capacity to manage an excess is smaller, the potential hazard of *in vivo* release of the metal ion seems likely to be much higher than for Fe^{3+}.

3.3 IRON OXIDE PARTICLES

Two categories of iron oxide particles have been described, differentiated exclusively by their size. Larger than 50 nm diameter iron oxide particles are classified as superparamagnetic iron oxide; smaller than 50 nm diameter they are classified as ultrasmall paramagnetic iron oxide. In the context of a contrast agent, the first thing to note is the massive size of these agents compared to the gadolinium chelates currently employed, which have a hydrodynamic diameter of around 10 Å. Inevitably, this means that they have very different pharmacokinetics. They are slow to extravasate; they are too large to clear from the body, being taken up by the cells of the immune system and the liver and eventually incorporated into the body's natural iron pool. This means that they can be excellent agents for iron replacement therapy, but it creates challenges for imaging. The difference in pharmacokinetics places limits on the timing of an imaging protocol in relation to the administration of the agent. A significant delay may need to be allowed for the agent to localize. Because the agent persists for a long time (~days), a follow-up imaging protocol is not possible for some time after administration. For a human with well-regulated iron levels, there is capacity in ferritin and hemoglobin to accommodate the additional iron provided by about two doses of an ultrasmall paramagnetic iron oxide. But one important lesson learned from the emergence of NSF is that providers often do not track or even know what agents a patient has been administered. Without adequate tracking, there is a possibility that a patient could be administered too many doses in a short space of time, creating iron overload.

Until now, without being explicit, we have discussed relaxivity exclusively in terms of longitudinal relaxivity, the effect on T_1. But all paramagnetic species will affect transverse relaxation (T_2 and T_2^*) as well as T_1. *In vivo*, T_2 is very short, much shorter than T_1. The transverse relaxivity of a low-molecular-weight chelate is too small to effect a large enough change on T_2 *in vivo*. The very large magnetic moment of an iron oxide particle means that not only do they shorten T_1 effectively, but they have even more profound effects on T_2 and T_2^*. It also means that their effects are not localized, and significant "blooming" can occur arising from the presence of these agents. T_2^* is the time constant for pure spin-spin relaxation summed with the contribution from local field inhomogeneities. The shortening of T_2 and T_2^* can be so profound that in T_1-weighted imaging, it may be difficult to eliminate their effects. These agents are most commonly used in T_2-weighted imaging protocols, in which they darken rather than brighten the image.

Iron oxide particles do not represent a potential like-for-like replacement of gadolinium agents, although they may have their place in MR imaging.

3.4 LOW MOLECULAR WEIGHT CHELATES

The chelates of high-spin d^5 transition metals face two significant challenges when it comes to developing contrast agents. The first of these is redox chemistry. To remain an effective relaxation agent a low molecular weight chelate must preserve the electronic configuration of the metal ion, so the first role of a ligand in a transition metal chelate must be to stabilize the oxidation state.

The second challenge concerns the robustness of the chelate. Transition metals have substantial ligand field effects that can stabilize a complex. A high-spin configuration is required and can be ensured by the simple expedient of avoiding strong field ligands. But in a high-spin configuration the electrons are distributed evenly between bonding and antibonding orbitals; meaning that there is no stabilization of the bonding interaction between metal and ligand from these electrons, according to Equation (3).

$$LFSE = (3 \times -0.4\Delta) + (2 \times 0.6\Delta) = 0 \qquad (2)$$

The required high-spin electronic configuration does not afford ligand field stabilization energy (LFSE) that could make the chelate more stable. This may seem disconnected from the real safety issue, namely kinetic robustness. But kinetics and thermodynamics are not quite as separate as we sometimes present them. The lower the energy (more thermodynamically stable) a chelate, the more potential there is for a larger activation energy to dissociation. So, while it is true that a stable chelate is not necessarily inert and *vice versa*, it is more likely that a chelate will be resistant to dissociation if it is more stable. Once more, robustness comes down to the strength of electrostatic interactions and in this context a smaller and more charge-dense metal ion is likely to be favored. Stable chelates of the charge dense Fe^{3+} are well-known and not only is Fe^{3+} more likely than Mn^{2+} to afford robust chelates; if Fe^{3+} is released in small quantities, it is less likely to cause severe problems than even a tiny amount of Mn^{2+}. Chelate robustness will also be influenced by other factors, such as ligand denticity and rigidity, which may assist in overcoming the absence of LFSE. How these factors are married with the other requirements of relaxation agent, time will tell. Perspectives on strategies for achieving this goal can be found in recent articles [32, 33].

It is instructive to consider the mode of action of MnDPDP, the only manganese chelate to enter clinical use as a contrast agent to date. In Gd^{3+} agents, the ligand is used to shield the metal ion from the biological milieu. The ligand in

MnDPDP served a very different purpose; it served the role of targeting vectors, causing the agent to preferentially accumulate in the liver and pancreas. It is notable that there are no coordinated water molecules in MnDPDP, and the intact complex does not serve as an effective relaxation agent. MnDPDP was specifically designed to release its Mn^{2+} ion to generate the aqua ion $(Mn(H_2O)_6)$, an effective relaxation agent. The packaging insert even provides clearance kinetics for intact chelate, ligand, and liberated Mn^{2+}. In this context, it is perhaps not surprising that the reasons for its withdrawal included safety concerns.

4   THE FUTURE OF GADOLINIUM IN MRI

We discuss here three potential future directions for gadolinium in the context of MRI. Both responsive and targeted contrast agents have been extensively reviewed previously, and it is not our intent to recapitulate these reviews here. Rather, we hope to provide perspective and context on the potential associated with each new direction.

4.1   RESPONSIVE AGENTS

Responsive contrast agents were first conceived by Meade and co-workers in 1997, when they developed a gadolinium chelate that changed its relaxivity in response to the activity of an enzyme (β-galactidase) [34]. This report spurred the development of a range of agents that change relaxivity in response to the presence (or absence) of a wide range of biomarkers for disease. A common target for these efforts were agents that could report extracellular pH. A pH-responsive agent developed by Sherry and co-workers [35] provides an instructive example of the potential and challenges of this approach. First reported in 1999, GdDOTA-4AmP exhibits a significant change in relaxivity over a physiologically relevant range (Figure 7). This pH response was eventually attributed to modulation of the second hydration sphere of the chelate by the phosphonate groups as they changed the protonation state with changing pH [36]. Relaxivity increases from about $3.5\,mM^{-1}s^{-1}$ at pH 9 to a maximum of almost $10\,mM^{-1}s^{-1}$ at pH 6 (Figure 7, dashed red line). This change in relaxivity, centered as it is around normal physiological pH (Figure 7, dashed green line), meant that this chelate was of considerable interest as a diagnostic tool. However, generating a pH map using this agent was a significant challenge. This is because contrast agents are not detected directly; what is measured is their effect on water. The magnitude of an agent's effect on water depends not only its relaxivity but also on its concentration (Equation 2).

$$\frac{1}{T_1} = r_1\,[Gd]$$
(3)

It follows from our earlier discussion on how image contrast is generated that in a T_1-weighted image signal intensity relates directly to the relaxation rate constant

(a)

GdDOTA-4AmP^{5-}

GdDOTP^{5-}

(b)

(c)

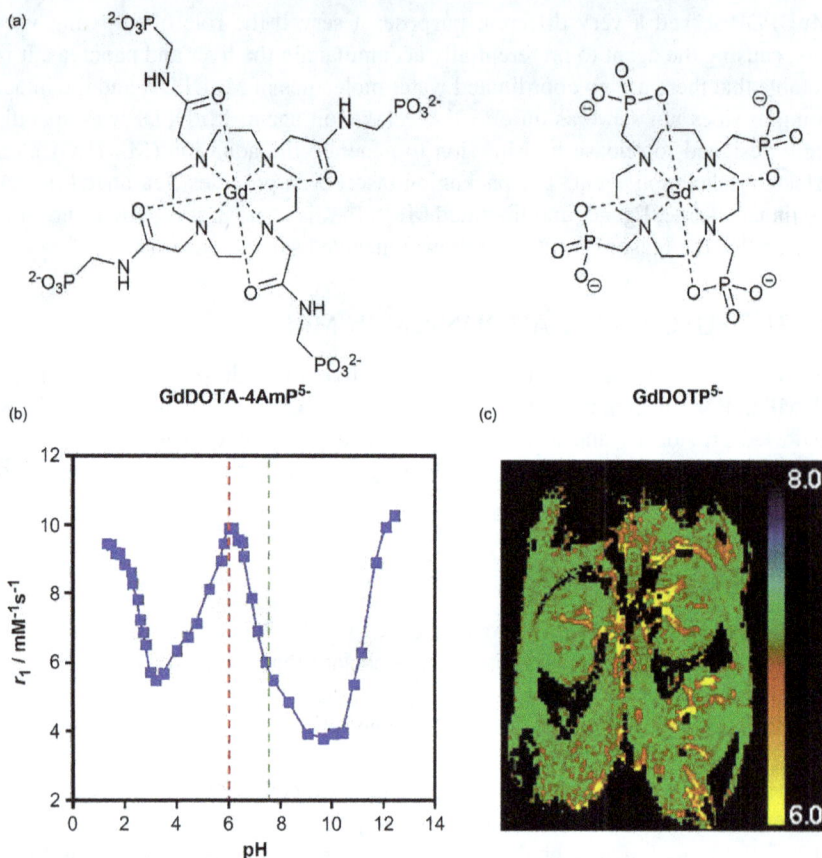

FIGURE 7   (a) The structures of GdDOTA-4AmP and GdDOTP. (b) The pH dependence of the relaxivity of GdDOTA-4AmP at 0.47 T and 25 °C. (c) A pH map of rat kidneys produced using GdDOTA-4AmP and GdDOTP.

$(1/T_1)$. In a contrast-enhanced image, this is determined by the product of the relaxivity and the agent's concentration, Equation (2). So, pH can be related to signal intensity through the relaxivity of the contrast agent, but only if the local concentration of the agent is known. But how is the local *in vivo* concentration of the agent to be determined if relaxivity is not constant? Gillies and co-workers came up with an ingenious solution to this seemingly intractable problem [37]. They used GdDOTP as a surrogate (Figure 7). GdDOTP is structurally similar to GdDOTA-4AmP: each is based on the same macrocyclic ring, each has four phosphonates, and each is pentaanionic, but the relaxivity of GdDOTP is not sensitive to pH. This means that GdDOTP could be administered and imaged using dynamic contrast-enhanced MRI methods; this would provide a baseline measurement of the change in agent concentration over time (based on Equation 2).

The assumption is made that the structural similarity between GdDOTP and GdDOTA-4AmP means that they have identical pharmacokinetics. So, when the dynamic contrast-enhanced MRI is repeated with GdDOTA-4AmP, concentration is used as the the known variable in Equation 2, allowing relaxivity to be extracted. Comparing with a calibration curve affords pH_e, the extracellular pH. In this way, Gillies and co-workers were able to generate pH maps first of the kidneys [37] and later of tumors [38,39].

This method is hardly a convenient method for producing a pH map. It requires the administration of two doses of contrast agents. In an era of heightened concern over the safety of gadolinium, a protocol that involves two consecutive doses of a contrast agent may not now be acceptable. A calibration curve is required. Figure 7 suggests that this is already in hand; however, because relaxivity is field dependent, a new calibration curve must be generated for every field at which the imaging is proposed.

There is also the viability of GdDOTA-4AmP as a clinical imaging agent to consider. It is well known that phosphonate groups have a strong affinity for calcium and that the primary storage location of Ca^{2+} is bone. Biodistribution studies on GdDOTA-4AmP show that just 2 hours after administration, more than 30% of the injected dose has accumulated in bone [40]. A similar affinity for bone is known for GdDOTP [41]. These results suggest that the clearance of these agents would be too slow.

4.2 TARGETED AGENTS

A target contrast agent is intended to selectively accumulate in tissue in which a specific biomarker of a disease is present in higher concentrations than normal tissue. In so doing, the affected region is expected to appear bright on an MR image. The development of practical targeted imaging agents must overcome three practical challenges: (1) the high detection limits of contrast agents, (2) the balance of specificity and pharmacokinetics, and (3) the economics of contrast agents.

4.2.1 Reducing Detection Limits

Clinical contrast agents are used at comparatively high doses (typically 0.1 mmolkg^{-1}). This is because clinically available contrast agents are comparatively inefficient – their relaxivities are comparatively low. The preceding discussion showed that gadolinium chelates could be made as much as 20 times more efficient. This goal would require simultaneous optimization of all the physiochemical parameters that govern relaxivity: r_{GdH}, τ_M, τ_R, and T_{1e} and T_{2e}. We will consider that the maximum permissible value of q is one so that the stability and safety of the chelate are preserved.

Attention has primarily focused on optimizing τ_M, in part because it is already known how to optimize τ_R. Conversely, the impact of coordination chemistry on electron spin relaxation was poorly understood, and rational strategies for optimizing T_{1e} and T_{2e} were difficult to develop. Many successful strategies for accelerating water exchange in gadolinium chelates have been reported [42,43], although sometimes at the expense of r_{GdH} [12,44]. Only recently has our own work yielded a chelate that, for the first time, simultaneously optimized all the parameters. GdDOTFA, when bound to human serum albumin (HSA), is the first chelate, to our knowledge, to exhibit maximum relaxivity – 110 mM^{-1}s^{-1} at 25°C and 0.47 T (Figure 8) [45]. This chelate provides a template from which agents with low detection limits can be obtained. However, excitement should be tempered by the recognition that this very high relaxivity is achieved at 0.47 T, a much lower field than is used in modern clinical imaging. As the field strength increases to 1.5 and 3.0 T in the fields currently in use in radiology, the maximum theoretical

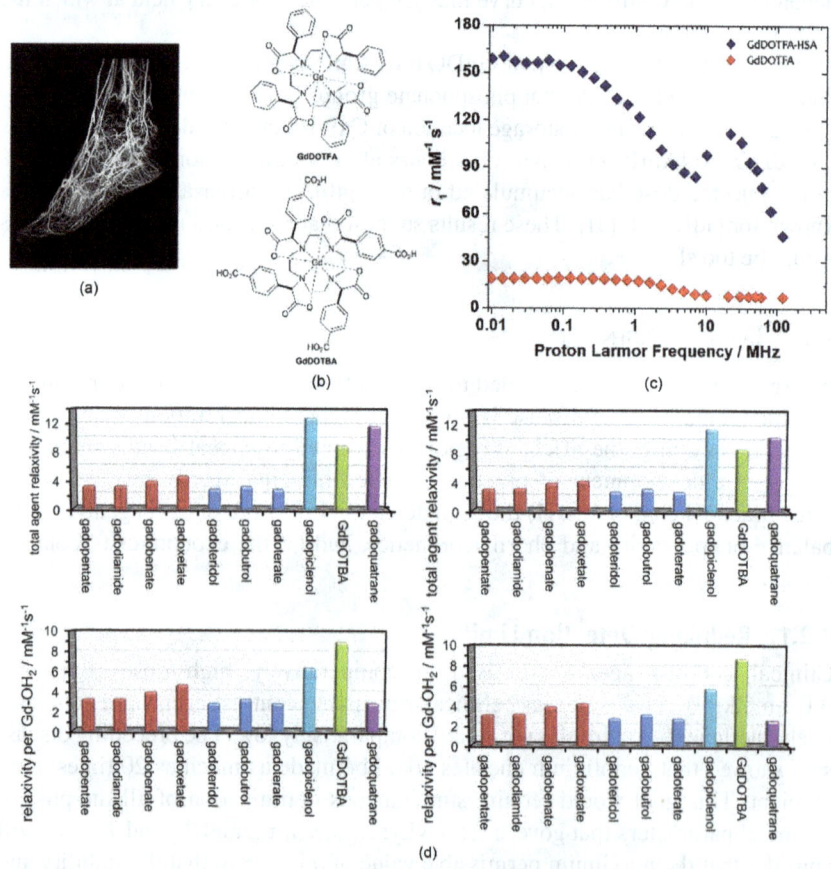

FIGURE 8   (a) An angiogram of a human foot acquired using MS-325. (b) The structures of GdDOTFA and GdDOTBA. (c) The Nuclear Magnetic Relaxation Dispersion profile of GdDOTFA (red diamonds) and of GdDOTFA when bound to HSA (blue diamonds) at 25 °C. (d) A comparison of the relaxivity of GdDOTBA at 37 °C with other available agents at 1.5 T (left) and 3.0 T (right).

relaxivity decreases markedly (Figure 8). GdDOTFA still performs excellently at higher fields, but its relaxivity drops off significantly (Figure 8). This will, to some extent, be offset by the fact that tissue T_1 increases with increasing field [46]. So detection limits will not drop as quickly as relaxivity; however, it does bring into question how low detection limits can be pushed in clinical imaging fields.

4.2.2   Limitations of Targeting Vectors

Developing a targeted agent means reconciling two competing demands: generating tissue specificity without preventing the agent from reaching the tissue. The entire premise of the agent rests on the idea that the agent will accumulate in the diseased tissue and only the diseased tissue [47]. So, it must incorporate a targeting vector that is highly selective for the target biomarker. Advances in biochemistry have made such highly selective vectors widely available. But if this targeting vector is very large, for example, an antibody fragment, then the agent may extravasate only slowly (if at all), potentially limiting its ability to reach the tissue it is intended to highlight. It may also clear slowly from the body, creating two potential problems. The most obvious of these is the potential safety risk associated with slow chelate clearance. But there is also a practical difficulty: extravasation will initially distribute non-selectively throughout tissue. The aim of the targeting vector is to retain the agent in diseased tissue while it clears from all the healthy tissue. But if clearance is slow, then a window for imaging in which the agent has accumulated in diseased tissue but is cleared from healthy tissue may not exist.

Ideally, a targeted contrast agent would function in the manner of the gadolinium-based contrast agent MS-325. It would have the properties of a low-molecular-weight chelate, including low relaxivity, until it binds to its target. At which point the increase in τ_R associated with binding will lead to a large increase in relaxivity, rendering the presence of an unbound agent unimportant.

4.2.3   Economic Challenges

The final challenge for a targeted agent is the high cost of regulatory approval and the slow rate of return on the investment. Only around one-third of MRI exams employ a contrast agent of any sort – a typical person may only receive one or two doses of a contrast agent in their lifetime. The market for contrast agents is small. The concept of the targeted agent makes this market even smaller. The currently available contrast agents are used to diagnose a wide variety of conditions. Once the use of the agent has become more and more specific, there will be fewer and fewer patients in need of that agent. Simply put, the economics of such an agent are unattractive. The targeting vector in the agent will need tissue specificity, which speaks to a complex structure that is difficult and expensive to produce. Production runs will be small because the number of patients requiring the agent will be small – this leads to high production costs. But the small number of patients means that sales will be slow, to counter this the price in likely to have to be increased to unsustainable levels. Could an agent that costs as much or more than the scan itself be marketed? It seems difficult to see how the cost of securing approval can be recouped once intellectual property protections expire.

The story of MS-325 (Figure 3) is illustrative of the problem. The concept of MS-325 was brilliant: a gadolinium chelate that binds to one of the most abundant proteins in the body: HSA. Because HSA is a ubiquitous transport protein in blood, it is an excellent target. It is easy for the contrast agent to access, it is easy to target with a simple hydrophobic group, and it is abundant (0.6 mM in serum). The binding of MS-325 to HSA has two beneficial effects: firstly, it slows the tumbling of the agent, increasing relaxivity; and secondly, it confines the agent to the blood pool. This means that astonishing images of the vasculature could be generated (Figure 8A) using lower doses (0.03 mmolkg^{-1}) than a conventional agent [48]. Epix and Schering won approval for MS-325 in various markets around 2006–2008. But initial sales of MS-325 were slow, and by the time Epix secured Food and Drug Administration approval in the United States, Schering pulled out of their joint marketing agreement [49]. In 2009, Epix sold the rights to MS-325 to Lantheus and went out of business [50]. If an agent targeted at an abundant protein like HSA struggles to make enough money, is there really a market for more narrowly tailored agents?

4.3   New Clinical Contrast Agents

In light of the previous discussion, it seems to us that the future of contrast agents does not involve either responsive or targeted agents. Nor does it seem likely that manganese- or iron-based agents are likely to breakthrough into the market either. This view is supported by recent developments. Two new agents, both based around gadolinium, have been developed [51,52]. The first of these, gadopiclenol, has recently received approval for clinical use and entered the marketplace. This chelate is unusual in that it disregards our earlier assumption that a chelate with more than one inner-sphere water molecule will not be sufficiently robust for *in vivo* use. Based around a different macrocycle (pyclen), the ligand is heptadentate, making this a $q=2$ chelate. Its relaxivity is correspondingly higher and further enhanced through the addition of molecular mass to the pendant arm, leading to a modest increase in τ_R. Relaxivity is 12.9 mM^{-1}s^{-1} at 37°C and 1.5 T and 11.6 mM^{-1}s^{-1} at 37°C and 3.0 T. This agent is now proposed for use at half the dose (0.05 mmolkg^{-1}) of other approved agents [53]. This should improve the safety profile of this agent without compromising performance (Figure 8D).

Another agent, gadoquatrane, is currently proceeding through phase III clinical trials. This agent is more conventional, relying on an octadentate macrocyclic ligation system. But unlike gadopiclenol, it includes four $q=1$ gadolinium ions, which increase molecular weight as well as adding paramagnetic centers. This means that the agent itself has high relaxivity: 47.2 mM^{-1}s^{-1} (37°C and 1.5 T) and 41.9 mM^{-1}s^{-1} (37°C and 3.0 T). Such high relaxivity is achieved by inclusion of four Gd^{3+} ions which renders the agent 2.4× more massive than current agents; the impact of the increased size remains to be seen. But by comparing relaxivity on a per Gd^{3+}-basis (11.8 mM^{-1}s^{-1} [37°C and 1.5 T] and 10.5 mM^{-1}s^{-1} [37°C and 3.0 T]) the impact of the increased size relative to gadopiclenol is apparent: the gadolinium in gadopiclenol is a more effective relaxation agent.

These developments point to the likely future of contrast agents in MRI: discrete chelates with high relaxivity – ideally with enhanced chelate stability – that permit lower doses with comparable performance. We have also been able to develop a discrete agent that has high relaxivity in imaging fields. GdDOTBA has relaxivities of $9.0\,mM^{-1}s^{-1}$ (37°C and 1.5 T) and $8.8\,mM^{-1}s^{-1}$ (37°C and 3.0 T) [43], slightly lower than those of gadopiclenol, but in this case the chelate $q = 1$. The gadolinium in GdDOTBA is optimized, affording exceptional performance of the gadolinium ion on a per-Gd-OH_2 basis (Figure 8D). It seems to us that chelates such as this, which can reduce the dose but remain safe, represent the future of contrast agents.

5   SUMMARY AND CONCLUSIONS

The future of gadolinium as the basis for contrast agents in MRI seems assured. Gadolinium-based agents continue to be widely used in clinical practice. And although there have been some high-profile problems with these agents, their safety profile continues to be very good. Few people suffer adverse reactions and if the best agents are used following best practices there is, for most patients, little to be concerned about. The problems with gadolinium agents most commonly occur in patients with renal insufficiency and this represents a group that continues to be underserved by options in diagnostic radiology. However, the increased awareness of the limitations of contrast agents that arose from the emergence of NSF in the 2000s means that greater attention is paid to following best practices.

The emergence of NSF has largely highlighted how valuable gadolinium is for diagnostic MRI; alternatives have failed to breakthrough, despite the intense interest in moving away from gadolinium. In our view, the 2010s may have been the "now or never" moment for Fe^{3+} and Mn^{2+}, and the chemistry of those agents did not step up to the challenge. In contrast, new higher relaxivity gadolinium chelates have been developed, with one example now available for clinical use. The higher relaxivity of these new agents should permit lower doses and improve safety for patients. The future of gadolinium appears bright.

ABBREVIATIONS AND DEFINITIONS

$1/T_{1e}$ **and** $1/T_{2e}$	electron spin relaxation rates (longitudinal and transverse)
$1/t_M$	water exchange rate
$1/t_R$	molecular tumbling rate
B_0	primary (applied) magnetic field
CN	coordination number
CT	computed tomography
D	ligand field splitting (magnitude of)
DOTA	2,2',2'',2''f'-(1,4,7,10-tetraazacyclododecane-1,4,7,10-tetrayl) tetraacetate
DTPA	diethylenetriamine pentaacetate
G4	generation 4 dendrimer

GdDO3A-Butrol	Gadobutrol
GdDTPA	Gadopentate
GdDTPA-BMA	Gadodiamide
GdDTPA-BMEA	Gadoversetamide
HSA	human serum albumin
ICP-MS	inductively coupled plasma – mass spectrometry
k_D	dissociation rate
K_{ML}	metal – ligand complex stability constant
LFSE	ligand field stabilization energy
MR	magnetic resonance
MRI	magnetic resonance imaging
M_{xy}	magnitude of magnetization in the transverse plane
M_Z	magnitude of magnetization along the longitudinal axis
NMR	nuclear magnetic resonance
NSF	nephrogenic systemic fibrosis
pH_e	extracellular pH
q	number of water molecules bound to metal ion
r	distance of the water molecule to the metal ion
r_1	relaxivity
r_{GdH}	relaxivity of the gadolinium-bound water proton
T_1	longitudinal relaxation time
T_2^*	time constant for pure spin-spin relaxation
T_2	transverse relaxation time
T_E	time between excitation pulse and peak of echo
T_R	time between successive excitation pulses

REFERENCES

1. F. Bloch, W. W. Hansen, M. Packard, *Phys. Rev.* **1946**, *69*, 127–127.
2. F. Bloch, *Phys. Rev.* **1946**, *70*, 460–474.
3. P. C. Lauterbur, *Nature*, **1973**, *242*, 190–191.
4. J. Keeler, *Understanding NMR Spectroscopy*, 2nd ed., John Wiley & Sons, New York, **2010**.
5. S. J. Lippard, J. M. Berg, *Principles of Bioinorganic Chemistry*, University Science Books, Mill Valley CA, **1994**.
6. A. D. Sherry, P. Caravan, R. E. Lenkinski, *J. Magn. Reson. Imaging*, **2009**, *30*, 1240–1248.
7. T. J. Clough, L. Jiang, K.-L. Wong, N. J. Long, *Nat. Commun.* **2019**, *10*, **1420**.
8. N. Sato, H. Kobayashi, A. Hiraga, T. Saga, K. Togashi, J. Konishi, M. W. Brechbiel, *Magn. Reson. Med.* **2001**, *46*, 1169–1173.
9. N. Bloembergen, *J. Chem. Phys.* **1957**, *27*, 572–573.
10. N. Bloembergen, L. O. Morgan, *J. Chem. Phys.* **1961**, *34*, 842–850.
11. I. Solomon, *Phys. Rev.* **1955**, *99*, 559–565.
12. B. C. Webber, M. Woods, *Dalton Trans.* **2014**, *43*, 251–258.
13. L. Banci, I. Bertini, C. Luchinat, *Inorganica Chim. Acta*, **1985**, *100*, 173–181.

14. M. R. Prince, H. Zhang, Z. Zou, R. B. Staron, P. W. Brill, *Am. J. Roentgenol.* **2011**, *196*, W138–W143.
15. M. R. Prince, C. Arnoldus, J. K. Frisoli, *J. Magn. Reson. Imaging*, **1996**, *6*, 162–166.
16. M. S. Nacif, A. E. Arai, J. A. Lima, D. A. Bluemke, *J. Cardiovasc. Magn. Reson.* **2012**, *14*, 18. doi: 10.1186/1532-429X-14-18. PMID: 22376193; PMCID: PMC3305456.
17. S. E. Cowper, L. D. Su, J. Bhawan, H. S. Robin, P. E. LeBoit, *Am. J. Dermatopathol.* **2001**, *23*, 383.
18. S. E. Cowper, *Curr. Opin. Rheumatol.* **2003**, *15*, 785–790.
19. S. E. Cowper, H. S. Robin, S. M. Steinberg, L. D. Su, S. Gupta, P. E. LeBoit, Lancet, **2000**, *356*, 1000.
20. D. Hao, T. Ai, F. Goerner, X. Hu, V. M. Runge, M. Tweedle, *J. Magn. Reson. Imaging*, **2012**, *36*, 1060–1071.
21. W. P. Cacheris, S. C. Quay, S. M. Rocklage, *Magn. Reson. Imaging*, **1990**, *8*, 467–481.
22. mriquestions.com/mn-agents-teslascan,   https://mriquestions.com/mn-agents-teslascan.html.
23. M. F. Tweedle, P. M. Wedeking, K. Kumar, *Invest. Radiol.* **1995**, *30*, 372–380.
24. P. Wedeking, M. Tweedle, *Int. J. Rad. Appl. Instrum. B*, **1988**, *15*, 395–402.
25. P. Wedeking, K. Kumar, M. F. Tweedle, *Magn. Reson. Imaging*, **1992**, *10*, 641–648.
26. T. Kanda, K. Ishii, H. Kawaguchi, K. Kitajima, D. Takenaka, *Radiology*, **2014**, *270*, 834–841.
27. K. A. Layne, K. Layne, D. M. Wood, P. I. Dargan, *Clin. Toxicol.* **2020**, *58*, 151–160.
28. H. Malikova, *Quant. Imaging Med. Surg.* **2019**, *9*, 1470–1474.
29. K. Y. Oh, V. H. J. Roberts, M. C. Schabel, K. L. Grove, M. Woods, A. E. Frias, *Radiology*, **2015**, *276*, 110–118.
30. M. F. Tweedle, *Invest. Radiol.* **2021**, *56*, 35–41.
31. https://hemochromatosis.org/
32. A. Gupta, P. Caravan, W. S. Price, C. Platas-Iglesias, E. M. Gale, *Inorg. Chem.* **2020**, *59*, 6648–6678.
33. P. Caravan, *Invest. Radiol.* **2024**, *59*, 187–196.
34. R. A. Moats, S. E. Fraser, T. J. Meade, *Angew. Chem. Int. Ed. Engl.* **1997**, *36*, 726–728.
35. S. Zhang, K. Wu, A. D. Sherry, *Angew. Chem. Int. Ed.* **1999**, *38*, 3192–3194.
36. F. K. Kálmán, M. Woods, P. Caravan, P. Jurek, M. Spiller, G. Tircsó, R. Király, E. Brücher and A. Dean. Sherry, *Inorg. Chem.*, **2007**, *46*, 5260–5270.
37. N. Raghunand, C. Howison, A. D. Sherry, S. Zhang, R. J. Gillies, *Magn. Reson. Med.* **2003**, *49*, 249–257.
38. M. L. Garcia-Martin, G. V. Martinez, N. Raghunand, A. D. Sherry, S. Zhang, R. J. Gillies, *Magn. Reson. Med.*, **2006**, *55*, 309–315.
39. G. V. Martinez, X. Zhang, M. L. Garcia-Martin, D. L. Morse, M. Woods, A. D. Sherry, R. J. Gillies, *NMR Biomed.* **2011**, *24*, 1380–1391.
40. M. Woods, P. Caravan, C. F. G. C. Geraldes, M. T. Greenfield, G. E. Kiefer, M. Lin, K. McMillan, M. I. M. Prata, A. C. Santos, X. Sun, J. Wang, S. Zhang, P. Zhao, A. Dean. Sherry, *Invest. Radiol.* **2008**, *43*, 861–870.
41. F. C. Alves, P. Donato, A. D. Sherry, A. M. Zaheer, S. Zhang, A. J. M. M. Lubag, M. E. Merritt, R. E. Lenkinski, J. V. Frangioni, M. Neves, M. I. M. Prata, A. C. Santos, J. J. P. de Lima, C. F. G. C. Geraldes, *Invest. Radiol.* **2003**, *38*, 750–760.
42. S. Avedano, L. Tei, A. Lombardi, G. B. Giovenzana, S. Aime, D. Longo, M. Botta, *Chem. Commun.* **2007**, 4726–4728.

43. M. Woods, Z. Kovacs, S. Zhang, A. D. Sherry, *Angew. Chem. Int. Ed.* **2003**, *42*, 5889–5892.
44. B. C. Webber, K. M. Payne, L. N. Rust, C. Cassino, F. Carniato, T. McCormick, M. Botta, M. Woods, *Inorg. Chem.* **2020**, *59*, 9037–9046.
45. K. B. Maier, L. N. Rust, F. Carniato, M. Botta and M. Woods, *Chem. Commun.*, **2024**, *60*, 2898–2901.
46. W. D. Rooney, G. Johnson, X. Li, E. R. Cohen, S.-G. Kim, K. Ugurbil, C. S. Springer, *Magn. Reson. Med.* **2007**, *57*, 308–318.
47. M. Woods, A. D. Sherry, *Chim. Oggi*, **2005**, *23*, 31–34.
48. bayer-schering-pharma/i/science-fuss-vasovist-presskit,c11743, https://news.cision.com/se/bayer-schering-pharma/i/science-fuss-vasovist-presskit,c11743.
49. 15587969/bayer-schering-epix-to-end-vasovist-partnership, https://www.auntminnie.com/clinical-news/interventional/article/15587969/bayer-schering-epix-to-end-vasovist-partnership.
50. 15591766/pharma-developer-epix-to-shut-down-liquidate-assets, https://www.auntminnie.com/clinical-news/interventional/article/15591766/pharma-developer-epix-to-shut-down-liquidate-assets.
51. J. Lohrke, M. Berger, T. Frenzel, C.-S. Hilger, G. Jost, O. Panknin, M. Bauser, W. Ebert, H. Pietsch, *Invest. Radiol.* **2022**, *57*, 629–638.
52. P. Robert, V. Vives, A.-L. Grindel, S. Kremer, G. Bierry, G. Louin, S. Ballet, C. Corot, *Radiology*, **2020**, *294*, 117–126.
53. M. Bendszus, D. Roberts, B. Kolumban, J. A. Meza, D. Bereczki, D. San-Juan, B. P. Liu, N. Anzalone, K. Maravilla, *Invest. Radiol.* **2020**, *55*, 129–137.

Index

Note: **Bold** page numbers refer to tables; *italic* page numbers refer to figures.

For Product Safety Concerns and Information please contact our EU
representative GPSR@taylorandfrancis.com
Taylor & Francis Verlag GmbH, Kaufingerstraße 24, 80331 München, Germany

www.ingramcontent.com/pod-product-compliance
Lightning Source LLC
Chambersburg PA
CBHW070722220326
41598CB00024BA/3258

9 781032 422169